Quality Systems and GMP Regulations for Device Manufacturers: A Practical Guide to U.S., European, and ISO Requirements

Also available from ASQ Quality Press

The FDA and Worldwide Quality System Requirements Guidebook for Medical Devices
Compiled by Kimberly A. Trautman

Product Development Planning for Health Care Products Regulated by the FDA
Elaine Whitmore

AAMI Quality System Standards Handbook for Medical Devices
Compiled by the Association for the Advancement of Medical Devices

Practical Product Assurance Management
John Bieda

CE-Mark: The New European Legislation for Products
SWBC, Organization for the European Conformity of Products

The Quality Audit Handbook
ASQ Quality Audit Division, J.P. Russell, editing director

Nimble Documentation®: The Practical Guide for World-Class Organizations
Adrienne Escoe

To request a complimentary catalog of ASQ Quality Press publications, call 800-248-1946.

Quality Systems and GMP Regulations for Device Manufacturers: A Practical Guide to U.S., European, and ISO Requirements

Steven S. Kuwahara

ASQ Quality Press
Milwaukee, Wisconsin

Interpharm Press
Buffalo Grove, Illinois

Quality Systems and GMP Regulations for Device Manufacturers: A Practical Guide to U.S., European, and ISO Requirements
Steven S. Kuwahara

Library of Congress Cataloging in Publication Data
Kuwahara, Steven S.
    Quality systems and GMP regulations for device manufacturers: a practical guide to U.S., European, and ISO requirements/by Steven S. Kuwahara.
        p. cm.
    Includes index.
    ISBN 0-87389-426-X
        1. Medical instruments and apparatus—Standards—United States. 2. Medical instruments and apparatus—Standards—Europe. 3. Medical instruments and apparatus industry—Law and legislation—United States. 4. Medical instruments and apparatus industry—Law and legislation—Europe. I. Title
KF3827.M4K893   1998
344.73'042—dc21   98-10632
                                                                                                                    CIP

© 1998 by ASQ Quality Press

10 9 8 7 6 5 4 3 2 1

ISBN 0-87389-426-X

Acquisitions Editor: Roger Holloway
Project Editor: Jeanne Bohn

ASQ Mission: To facilitate continuous improvement and increase customer satisfaction by identifying, communicating, and promoting the use of quality principles, concepts, and technologies; and thereby be recognized throughout the world as the leading authority on, and champion for, quality.

Attention: Schools and Corporations
ASQ Quality Press books, audiotapes, videotapes, and software are available at quantity discounts with bulk purchases for business, educational, or instructional use. For information, please contact ASQ Quality Press at 800-248-1946, or write to ASQ Quality Press, P.O. Box 3005, Milwaukee, WI 53201-3005.

For a free copy of the ASQ Quality Press Publications Catalog, including ASQ membership information, call 800-248-1946, or access http://www.asq.org.

Printed in the United States of America

 Printed on acid-free paper

American Society for Quality

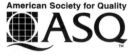

Quality Press
611 East Wisconsin Avenue
Milwaukee, Wisconsin 53202
Call toll free 800-248-1946
http://www.asq.org

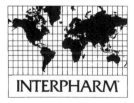

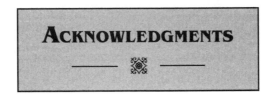

ACKNOWLEDGMENTS

A great big thank you to Sara and Dan and especially Rene for their support, which has been largely responsible for the completion of this work.

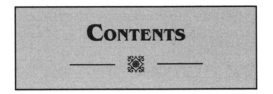

CONTENTS

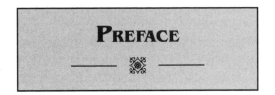

PREFACE

This book is intended for the company that is new to the world of device GMPs and ISO standards. It is designed to show QA/QC/RA workers how a quality system may be constructed to (1) comply with the U.S. Quality System regulations and (2) comply with the European standards that will lead to ISO registration. Part I is a general discussion of the documentation system that will be required and the Quality System regulations. Part II describes documents or classes of documents that need to be prepared to comply with the Quality System regulations. Part III compares the Quality System regulations with those developed by the ISO and other European regulators to show what additional documents need to be added to the Quality System regulations to meet the European device standards.

The original text, *Practical Guide to GMPs for Device and Diagnostic Manufacturers* (Interpharm Press 1997) was the result of a presentation made to a company that was in the early stages of product development. At this time there was a faction within the company that felt they should enter the European market, but feared this would be too costly because of the additional regulations that they would need to meet. In response to this internal debate, a document was prepared to show how much additional work would be required to produce a Quality System that would be capable of satisfying the requirements of the U.S. CGMP and ANSI/ISO/ASQC 9001:1994. Around this time, the FDA announced their intent to issue a final draft of the revised device GMPs that incorporated material originally contained in the ANSI/ISO/ASQC 9001:1994. Consequently, the job became one of advising the client on how to meet the new U.S. GMPs. This was initially done using a draft of the proposed CGMPs, and it became clear that because of the incorporation of the requirements from the ANSI/ISO/ASQC 9001:1994 into 21 CFR 820, the job of meeting ISO standards while complying with U.S. CGMPs was greatly simplified. Before my first book was printed, the final version of the new CGMPs was reviewed to ensure that no changes were required.

CDRH published guidelines to aid companies in meeting the requirements of the new CGMPs. The guidelines on Design Control and Risk Management were reviewed and, where applicable, incorporated into this book. Since then, additional material has been reviewed. These were ANSI/AAMI/ISO 13485:1996 which is based on ANSI/ISO/ASQC 9001 and provides more specific directions for manufacturers of medical devices. In this role it may replace EN 46001, which it closely approximates. In this second book, only a small amount of material refers to ANSI/AAMI/ISO 13485:1996, since EN 46001 already covered most of the material that is supplemental to ANSI/ISO/ASQC 9001. A second document which is more applicable for U.S.-based manufacturers is entitled "Medical Device Quality Systems Manual: A small entity compliance guide." First edition, December 1996 (HHS Publication FDA 97-4179). This Quality Systems Manual may be obtained from CDRH (DSMA). The Quality Systems Manual provides several examples or templates for forms and other documents that are very useful for specific situations and also provides detailed instructions for certain situations or regulations. However, many situations will require a more general approach which I hope to present in this book by taking an overview of the regulations so that the manufacturer may decide on what is appropriate for its particular product.

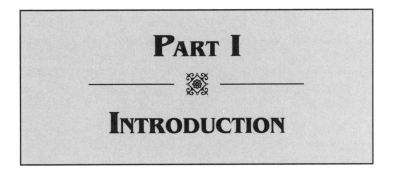

PART I

INTRODUCTION

The following discussion is presented to aid the device manufacturer in preparing the documentation necessary to comply with the provisions of the newly adopted device Current Good Manufacturing Practices (CGMP) (21 CFR 820, effective June 1, 1997) which are also being called the Quality System regulations. Not all of the CGMPs are really new, so a part of what is presented here should cover documents already existing at the manufacturer's facility. The problem, of course, is which documents? Each manufacturer has its own unique needs and approach to documentation so a presentation aimed at exact needs cannot be done. Consequently, this book approaches the subject from the point of view of a new company with no preexisting documentation. In this way, companies that already have documents in place may ignore redundant subjects, while new manufacturers or manufacturers new to the medical device industry will receive a detailed coverage of the CGMPs and the documents that may be generated in the course of meeting their requirements.

Coverage of the CGMPs cannot guarantee that the manufacturer will successfully pass a U.S. Food and Drug Administration (FDA) inspection the first time out. Inspectors vary in their personal interpretations and attitudes toward the importance of the various CGMP sections and in the manner that they would like to see problems handled. It also appears that the agency periodically targets certain

1

areas for in-depth coverage. This may be the result of FDA policy changes or due to training courses, but the manufacturer must realize that emphasis does change.

This book only gives one person's approach, which is not necessarily the FDA's approach. Also, each manufacturer is different and has its own way of looking at a subject. In some cases, different manufacturers may have documents that are so dissimilar that one wonders if they are both reading the same regulation. Some manufacturers have documents that completely miss the point of a regulation. In fact, some even have documents in which the body of the document does not cover the subject of the title.

Remember that the documentation system does not confer quality on the product. It can only guide and direct. The world's greatest documentation system cannot make a product. The manufacturer's employees, from top management to the janitorial staff, must assume responsibility for executing the directions and following the spirit of the regulations. The manufacturer with the "do what we need to get by" attitude will produce a device that "gets by," but it will not be of the best quality that the manufacturer is capable of attaining. A company's quality system is usually a reflection of the attitude of the company's upper management toward quality. The time, effort, and funds needed to produce a properly functioning quality system are such that strong upper management commitment is needed to have a truly successful program. All too often, upper management talks enthusiastically about quality, while audits and inspections reveal a quality system that is deprived of funds and managerial support. Neither slogans nor advertising will make a quality product. Products are made by people, and people will do what they feel their management wants them to do. If the advertising talks about quality, but the orders on the shop floor are to "do what you need to do to get the product out the door," the product will suffer along with employee morale.

※ Current Good Manufacturing ※ Practices (CGMPs)

Part II of this book covers the device CGMPs found in part 820 of title 21 of the Code of Federal Regulations (21 CFR 820), now known as the Quality System regulations. There are other CGMPs. These are CGMPs for the manufacture of foods (21 CFR 110) or for drugs and biologics (21 CFR 210 and 211) with special CGMPs for blood and its components (21 CFR 606), and special general regulations for biologics (21 CFR 610) and *in vitro* diagnostics (21 CFR 809). In addition there are other parts of title 21 that affect the manufacturer of medical devices, especially 21 CFR 803, 807, 808 and 812. These are parts dealing with licensing, importation, adverse event reporting, and so on. If the device works with a biologic or drug, other requirements will come into play. Some of these parts of the CFR will be mentioned in the discussion of how sections of these CGMPs interact with the other parts of the regulations. Part 820 is important, because it addresses the manufacturer's quality system. The new revision of part 820 incorporates elements of the International Organization for Standardization (ISO) 9001 standard, making it easier for a manufacturer to meet CGMP and ANSI/ISO/ASQC 9001 requirements with one quality system.

The reader should note that the terms: CGMP, 21 CFR 820, and QS regulations are used interchangeably in this book. This is the result of the author being originally trained as a "GMP person." In actuality, the term "QS regulations" is becoming more popular and serves the useful function of distinguishing the medical device GMP from the GMP for drugs and biologics. Note that the abbreviation QSR is not used because it can lead to confusion between QS regulations, QS records (defined as QSR in reference to 21 CFR 820.186), and QS requirements.

Part III discusses additional documents necessary for a company to comply with ANSI/ISO/ASQC 9001 after first meeting the requirements of the CGMP. In this regard the reader should review EN 46001 and ANSI/AAMI/ISO 13485:1996 which are European documents that cover the application of ANSI/ISO/ASQC 9001 to medical devices. The CGMP of 21 CFR 820, even in its newly revised form, is not identical to ANSI/ISO/ASQC 9001, so other documents or modifications to existing documents will be required. The additional documents are not unusually difficult to produce, and there really is no technical barrier to taking the extra steps to secure ISO registration. Part III is designed to allow a manufacturer to see what additional work is required to attain registration under the ANSI/ISO/ASQC 9001 standards. The manufacturer seeking registration under

ANSI/ISO/ASQC 9002 or 9003 can simply ignore the sections that do not apply. Part III was written with the U.S. manufacturer in mind, and the reader should be warned that simply reversing the requirements for a company already compliant with ANSI/ISO/ASQC 9001 may not work. In some cases, the CGMP requirement goes beyond the ISO standard in a way that compliance with the CGMP will cover the ISO standard, but the ISO standard may not meet all of the requirements of the QS regulations.

Meeting CGMPs will not protect the company from competition based on quality. The competitor who goes the extra step for quality without causing the customer to incur a significant cost penalty will gain a marketing advantage that may be insurmountable. Also, the company may make claims that exceed the minimums imposed by the QS regulations. In this case, the company will need to take steps to ensure the production of a product that meets the higher standards. The QS regulation must be regarded as basic requirements that must be met so the public (in the form of the FDA) will feel assured that the device is safe and efficacious.

❖ Documentation System ❖

This book discusses documents and the methods used to classify, store, retrieve, and prepare documents that are critical to the proper operation of the quality system and the company in general. The documentation system proposed here is a company-wide system with the responsibility for documents from all parts of the company. The documents themselves will be generally applicable to the whole company. If a document is prepared by one group, other groups should be free to use it in their operations. A product specification written by a development team can be used as a reference by the testing group and as a purchasing specification by the purchasing department. Companies that have individual departmental document systems are usually confronted with conflicting documents, general confusion, frustrated supervisors, and fed-up employees.

The basic need is to have everything written down. Civil servants have long had a saying that, "if it isn't in a memo; it doesn't exist," and the wise manufacturer will adopt a similar policy. The documentation will provide long-term continuity as employees come and go and technology changes. The documentation will tie parts of the company together and provide coordinating mechanisms, so that different departments and divisions can work together in concert, rather than conflict. The documents will provide the basis for training programs so that a new hire can rapidly learn the basics of the job and, hopefully, some of the tricks of the trade. The documents are records that will provide information on what has gone before and which mistakes do not need to be repeated. The need is to document and record the activities of the company so that everyone can work from the same knowledge base. The documentation system described here should incorporate the requirements that are distributed throughout 21 CFR 820 and not be just concerned with the needs of 21 CFR 820.40 and Subpart M.

The documentation system most often described as meeting the ISO requirements uses a multitiered stratification that defines the relationship among documents. This stratification is useful for both ISO and CGMP documentation needs and is useful even if the manufacturer has no intention of seeking ISO registration. The 1987 version of ANSI/ISO/ASQC 9001 divides documents into the Quality Manual (QM), Procedures, Work Instructions, and Records, in that order. The system is often described as a pyramid, with the QM at the apex and the Records as the broad base. The width of each band is designed to show the number of documents in each stratum. The 1994 version of ANSI/ISO/ASQC 9001 combined Work Instructions and Procedures to produce a pyramid of three tiers, showing QM, Procedures, and Records. Working down the pyramid, each level of documents should lead to the one below it. Policies lead to Procedures, which lead to Work Instructions, and, finally, Records. Despite the change in 1994, it is still useful for the manufacturer to think of documents in four tiers (perhaps Work Instructions could be known as Type B Procedures). Consider the following example based on process validations.

> *The QM document would be a policy statement that contains general procedural statements. For instance, it might say that processes shall be validated; the following types of processes are to be validated; validations shall employ statistical methods; they shall be performed by the following organizations on three consecutive production runs; all routine testing shall be performed;*

statistical analysis shall be done on the results to show homogeneity among the runs; the validation study report shall be reviewed. There would then be procedural documents and work instructions. In general, procedures give general instructions on "how to . . ." while work instructions are directions that are specific to the particular instance. The procedures would be documents such as scheduling procedures, procedures for Statistical Process Control, procedures for analytical testing, or procedures for statistical analysis. A major work instruction here would be the "Run Sheets for the Validation of the . . . Process." The procedures could lead to or be replaced by Work Instructions. In most cases, Work Instructions are a step-by-step series of directions for accomplishing a particular process. They represent the application of the policy and procedural documents to the current process. The variety of Work Instructions known as run sheets *usually has blanks or check off boxes to record data or the results of actions and are records as well as procedures. The final level of documents includes records such as filled-in run sheets, the validation study report, the test result forms, the statistical analysis sheets, and lot release documents.*

Note that this example describes a system in which the documents appear to run in a top-down fashion. In some cases, for instance when designing a new documentation system for compliance with ISO or CGMP requirements, it will be found that working from the bottom up is better, because many companies, even small companies just beginning, already have Records and Work Instructions. These could then be grouped, missing documents noted and prepared, and the system could be built up to the Quality Manual. It is much better to have Work Instructions and Records without a Quality Manual than vice versa.

If a company has a set of documents, it is critical for everyone to follow those instructions. If a company is weak in following its own documents (and there are many symptoms of this), an auditor or inspector can have a field day generating observations and findings by interviewing people on the manufacturing line or in the testing laboratories. Worse yet, a company can have a serious breakdown in its internal communications that will, in turn, produce chaotic conditions on its manufacturing lines. A major problem can arise from the use of "redlined" documents. These are documents that have undergone a local change through the expedience of crossing out words and writing in the desired instructions (using a red ink pen). This procedure is fine if the redline is a one time occurrence and is quickly resolved by changing all copies of that document. The problem arises when the document is not rapidly updated, and the company has two or more groups using what are essentially different documents (the original document and the redlined document). This can easily lead to a chaotic situation where, for instance, different departments that have the same instrument use different calibration procedures. Some companies do not allow redlining, but insist that these changes must be handled as a deviation that must be resolved rapidly. However it is done, company management must ensure that documentation rules are enforced.

One frequently heard management response to the need to follow documentation is, "Well, if they're going to hold us to our documents, we just won't have a document." The problem is that there is one time when a manufacturer does need to have everything written down, and that is in the license application. No matter what the product, if the manufacturer is concerned with these CGMPs, there will, eventually, be a license application submitted to the FDA. Major problems can develop later if it is found that the workers assembling the device are not following the procedures that the Regulatory Affairs department thought were in use. With regard to records, juries are not very sympathetic to oral testimony unsupported by documentation, especially if the regulations say that records should have been maintained. The author has encountered situations where key employees have left work one evening and either never returned or did not return for months. In one instance, it was found that a key preparation step for a component had never been entirely written down. The one employee who knew the step was involved in an accident that left him in a coma. After he came out of the coma, it was necessary to interview the employee in his hospital bed so that his assistant could begin to duplicate his work. In another case, it was found that the only functional diagram of a large company's Water for Injection distribution system was in an employee's brain when she died in an automobile accident. When one considers the money and time involved with the operations of a plant, only a foolish manufacturer will attempt to use a system that depends on individual human memory.

The manufacturer should choose a good electronic data and document management system with an associated word processor that has wide compatibility. The ability to exchange files throughout the company and even with the FDA is an important consideration (computer-assisted submissions have been made to the FDA). In this day and age, there is no excuse for a documentation system based on paper hard copies alone. Paper copies can still be distributed, and in some instances have definite advantages, but the use of electronic media during the review and approval stages can greatly shorten the time needed for these activities, provided that document security systems are carefully designed. Similarly, the exchange of information among departments and divisions can be done electronically. Also, a word processor compatible with databases and spreadsheets will greatly aid in dealing with statistical procedures and monitoring activities required by the QS regulation.

The security system should be designed to limit employee access to documents not related to their work. Document classification is important for this and the classification system must be carefully designed to produce packets of closely related documents. All employees should be granted "read only" or "read and print only" access to all documents related to their work. Supervisors should have access to a wider range of documents, commensurate with their work requirements. Supervisors could also be granted "read, print, or copy to disk" access. Higher level supervisors would be granted access to a wider range of documents. Quality Assurance, Quality Control, and Regulatory Managers, and upper management would have access to all documents. All employees should be able to prepare new documents or modify existing documents, using a secondary memory location, such as floppy disks or a partition in the main memory unit. The ability to actually introduce a new document into the system or to change an existing document should be restricted to supervisory employees in the document control group, and these employees should be allowed to act only after review and approval of the new documents or changes have occurred.

The supervisor of the documentation system should have skills in word processing and with the spreadsheet and database that the company uses. This supervisor or an assistant should also be a skilled technical writer, capable of rewriting documents before they are entered into the documentation system. A large percentage of business school graduates, scientists, and engineers are very poor writers, and it is important to translate their documents into language that is easily understood by others. During auditing expeditions, the author has seen documents that were barely intelligible, having been written in bureaucratese with innumerable undefined abbreviations and acronyms. The problem is that poorly written documents are virtually useless for disseminating information or knowledge. Poorly written documents lead to unnecessary confusion and conflict and often invite deliberate misinterpretation. When one considers the cost of having documents prepared and maintained, it is silly to have an ineffective system. A company needs to protect itself by adopting uniform writing standards, including spelling. This can be done easily and inexpensively by adopting company dictionaries (regular collegiate and a medical dictionary) and specifying a trade or scientific journal for matters of style and usage. Trade journals often have a more uniform style than scientific journals. Basically, the procedure will state that if a certain style or usage can be found in the journal, it is acceptable for the manufacturer's documents. The company dictionary will serve as the reference for spelling and definitions. Since it is often difficult to have departments police their own documents, this function should be performed by documentation system personnel, who have clear instructions and authority to reject a poorly written document such as those with poor grammar, many misspelled words, or those that do not follow the company's template for the particular type of document.

The documents must be understandable by those who will be using them. Therefore, it may be necessary to ensure that certain documents be written at a secondary school level while others may be written at the undergraduate level. If circumstances dictate it, bilingual documents may be needed. If the work force is bilingual, the employer must take effective steps to train and inform all employees, and not hold to some rigid standard that can induce errors or misunderstanding. Some countries have laws which state that work instructions or employee rules must be written in the local language. Companies with international operations should check on these requirements. Also, the how-to documents should be written so that they can be followed by anyone with a general training in the field. This may mean that the documents must be very simplistic and written in a cookbook style. This is fine. It is better to be too detailed in the instructions than to have insufficient detail. Clear and detailed examples should be given for solving particular problems, including details on how the information is to be gathered, how the problem or equation is to be solved, and what is to be done with the final result. While people often make fun of U.S. Army training manuals, they miss the point. The Army needs to prepare documents that can be read and followed by personnel who may have limited reading skills. It does a manufacturer no good to have elegantly written documents that cannot be understood by its workers. The point is to inform and train workers, not to win writing prizes.

Standard document formats also need to be adopted for each type of document. This will greatly ease working with databases and will actually help with document preparation and retrieval. It should be easy to identify a particular paragraph or passage in a document, and one of the standard outline formats can be used. Each document should have a keyword list to aid in searches. It should have a unique document number and a date of issue so that revisions can be separated from each other.

Every document should be under some sort of control to prevent it from being revised without the knowledge and approval of management and the people who prepared the original document. At a minimum, it should be considered an act of common courtesy to allow a document's originator to have a say in its revision. Any document that can be changed and revised at will by any employee should be considered a memo and not made into a part of the documentation system.

All documents should be periodically reviewed to see if they reflect current practice. Auditing can be used to check on whether or not procedures are being followed, but auditing usually can only check a sample of currently active documents. Periodic reviews must be conducted to ensure that obsolete documents are purged from the system and archived. It is not useful to have, still in the system, detailed instructions on how to use a particular instrument five years after the instrument was sent to the recycling bin. An obsolete document is a waste of space or electronic memory. The usual way to handle this is to have documents sent back to the manager of the area that generated them with an attached memo asking if the document may be considered obsolete.

Obsolescence is usually based on the age of the documents. In some companies this is as short as two years while others only check on documents that are five years old. If the manager does not consider the document obsolete, the document should be checked against current practice and reissued with a new effective date. In this way the document will keep up with manufacturing practices as they evolve. The process for making a document obsolete or reissuing an existing one should follow the same approval process as the acceptance of a new document. This is important because it acts as a general notice and insures that all concerned agree with the decision to discard or reissue a document. The manufacturer will frequently find that a document considered obsolete by the issuing department is actually in current use by another. In these cases document ownership should be transferred to the other department and the document reissued. Similarly, when a document is being reissued, all user departments should be allowed to have some input on the acceptability of the document that is being reissued.

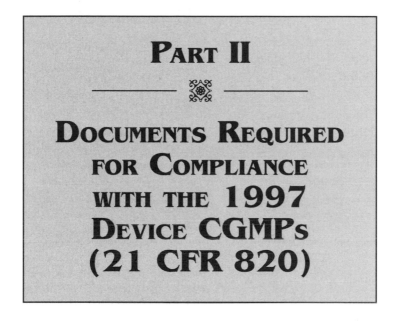

Part II

Documents Required for Compliance with the 1997 Device CGMPs (21 CFR 820)

Part II describes the files or documents that must be prepared and maintained for compliance with the device CGMPs in 21 CFR 820. In general, each file or document required by the regulations is set up as follows:

1. Title of the relevant section or paragraph.
2. Quotation (in italics) of the applicable passage from the device CGMP.
3. A numerical designation and a descriptive title of the document or file that should be prepared in response to the regulation.
4. A description and discussion of the contents of the required documents or file.

Not all of the documents discussed here are required. The manufacturer's structure and existing internal procedures will have a major impact on deciding the documentation needs of the company. Also, some sections contain suggestions for additional documents or the manufacturer may decide to divide a single document into more than one. The documentation system must fit the needs of the manufacturer. Consequently, the manufacturer must realize that what follows should not be taken as a rigid checklist that does not allow any variations or departures. Instead, the manufacturer should look upon the recommendations as guidelines that will help in attaining compliance.

For those who are new to the regulations and the FDA, it should be noted that the phrase 21 CFR 820.30 stands for "Title 21, Code of Federal Regulations, part 820, paragraph 30." For the sake of brevity, in situations where paragraphs or subparagraphs are not further designated, the reader should assume that they are included in the section that is cited. Thus 21 CFR 820.4 will include all paragraphs and subparagraphs such as 21 CFR 820.4(a), and 21 CFR 820.4(b) or 21 CFR 820.4(a)(1) as the case may be.

The documents that create, describe, and maintain the files or documents required by the device CGMP will tend to be high level documents. When dealing with the requirements of ANSI/ISO/ASQC 9001, these high-level documents should form the company quality manual. All of these documents along with the secondary documents that they create should then be regarded as quality system documents and be subject to change control. The documents listed as belonging to a file or set do not always need to be in that set. In some cases, the regulations state that a particular document should be in a particular file, but most documents have no specifications as to their grouping, and the manufacturer is free to classify the documents in a manner appropriate to the local operation. Other documents given in the book will be placed in a certain file or set because they appear to be related or because they were classified in such a manner by some organizations that the author has visited. Some documents will create a class of other documents, such as records of tests or instrument calibrations. These secondary documents may need to be placed in separate files of their own.

Because of the variations among company management styles and the large variety of items that are called medical devices, it is not possible to prepare a single list of documents that will be applicable in all cases. Sometimes, particular documents will be unnecessary due to the nature of the product or the internal structure of the company. In other cases, a company (especially a small company) may decide to combine two or more documents into a single procedure, while in others, the complexity of the device may force a company to create several documents to accomplish a processing step.

Where the author feels that a document or class of documents is needed, a number has been assigned to the document or the controlling document, and this will be shown next to the paragraph that describes it. For some sections, a document is not needed to satisfy the regulation. The regulation may be simply informing the reader that a certain thing is permissible, or not, or it may be stating the government's position on a certain point. In these cases, a comment may be made, but a document number will not be shown before the first paragraph of the discussion.

※ Subpart A—General Provisions ※

21 CFR 820.1 Scope

21 CFR 820.1(a) Applicability. **(1)** *Current good manufacturing practice (CGMP) requirements are set forth in this quality system regulation. The requirements in this part govern the methods used in, and the facilities and controls used for, the design, purchasing, manufacture, packaging, labeling, storage, installation, and servicing of all finished devices intended for human use. The regulations in this part are intended to ensure that finished devices will be safe and effective and otherwise in compliance with the Federal Food, Drug, and Cosmetic Act (the act). This part establishes basic requirements applicable to manufacturers of finished medical devices. If a manufacturer engages in only some operations subject to the requirements in this part, and not in others, that manufacturer need only comply with those requirements applicable to the operations in which it is engaged. With respect to class I devices, design controls apply only to those devices listed in § 820.30(a)(2). This regulation does not apply to manufacturers of components or parts of finished devices, but such manufacturers are encouraged to use appropriate provisions of this regulation as guidance. Manufacturers of human blood and blood components are not subject to this part, but are subject to part 606 of this chapter.*

(2) *The provisions of this part shall be applicable to any finished device and component described above, as defined in this part, intended for human use, that is manufactured, imported, or offered for import in any State or Territory of the United States, the District of Columbia, or the Commonwealth of Puerto Rico.*

(3) *In this regulation the term "where appropriate" is used several times. When a requirement is qualified by "where appropriate," it is deemed to be "appropriate" unless the manufacturer can document justification otherwise. A requirement is "appropriate" if nonimplementation could reasonably be expected to result in the product not meeting its specified requirements or the manufacturer not being able to carry out any necessary corrective action.*

It is not necessary to prepare a document to meet the requirements of 21 CFR 820.1(a), as it only contains general information. It does, however, mention three points of importance for CGMP reviews. First, not all class I devices are subject to design control, and manufacturers of the exempt devices may avoid most of the requirements of 21 CFR 820.30. However, these manufacturers may still be required to meet the standards of ANSI/ISO/ASQC 9001, instead of just those of ANSI/ISO/ASQC 9002, if they should seek ISO registration.

Second, manufacturers of components or parts do not need to meet CGMP requirements. However, the FDA suggests that manufacturers of components may wish to follow appropriate parts of the CGMP as guidance. Also, the primary manufacturer is still responsible for assuring that its suppliers, contractors, and consultants provide quality products. This requirement is covered under 21 CFR 820.50. The exemption is useful because it relieves the manufacturer from having to review or confirm the CGMP compliance status of suppliers of items such as small parts, paint, or light bulbs. At the same time, the manufacturer will want to carefully monitor a supplier of a critical component to ensure that the needed level of quality will continue to be met. Just because the supplier does not need to meet CGMP requirements, it does not mean that the manufacturer is obligated to purchase material that does not meet the manufacturer's specifications. If the manufacturer wishes to write specifications or even a requirement for GMP compliance into its purchasing contracts, it has the right to do so and to negotiate with the supplier over the requirements for the quality of the material.

If a component is an accessory to a finished device and is labeled and sold separately from the finished device, the component itself may be considered to be a finished device and be subject to licensing and the CGMP (21 CFR 807.20(a)(5)). For instance, a disposable tubing set that is designed to be integrated into a device, but which is also sold separately from the device, might require a license of its own. Therefore the act of simply declaring an item to be a component does not relieve the manufacturer of the component from CGMP requirements. In any case, the manufacturer of the finished device is always responsible for the quality of the device, and therefore needs to control the quality of its components.

Third, FDA has provided a definition of the term "where appropriate." There was much concern over varying interpretations of this term, and this definition helps. Basically, it says that a requirement is "appropriate" if it helps to maintain or improve the quality of a product. If a company decides that a regulation is "not appropriate," it should prepare and submit a report explaining the decision and justifying the action. At a minimum, the report should show that noncompliance with the regulation will not prevent a device from meeting specifications or result in a failure of the company to perform a necessary corrective action.

21 CFR 820.1(b) Limitations. *The quality system regulation in this part supplements regulations in other parts of this chapter except where explicitly stated otherwise. In the event that it is impossible to comply with all applicable regulations, both in this part and in other parts of this chapter, the regulations specifically applicable to the device in question shall supersede any other regulations.*

21 CFR 820.1(c) Authority. *Part 820 is established and promulgated under authority of sections 501, 502, 510, 513, 514, 515, 518, 519, 520, 522, 701, 704, 801, and 803 of the act (21 U.S.C. 351, 352, 360, 360c, 360d, 360e, 360h, 360i, 360j, 360l, 371, 374, 381, and 383). The failure to comply with any applicable provision in this part renders the device adulterated under section 501(h) of the act. Such a device, as well as any person responsible for the failure to comply, is subject to regulatory action under sections 301, 302, 303, 304, and 801 of the act.*

Paragraphs 21 CFR 820.1(b) and(c) mainly contain information of interest to the manufacturer's lawyers, and a document does not need to be prepared in response to them. One point to be noted here is that the people responsible for a device being noncompliant are also subject to regulatory action. This regulatory action can take the form of administrative (by FDA), civil, or criminal prosecution. In its response to comments on the Working Draft, the FDA noted that violations of the regulations do not need to be intentional to create a public health risk or for the FDA to take regulatory action.

21 CFR 820.1(d) Foreign Manufacturers. *If a manufacturer who offers devices for import into the United States refuses to permit or allow the completion of an FDA inspection of the foreign facility for the purpose of determining compliance with this part, it shall appear for purposes of section 801(a) of the act, that the methods used in, and the facilities and controls used for, the design, purchasing, manufacture, packaging, labeling, storage, installation, or servicing of any devices produced at such facility that are offered for import into the United States do not conform to the requirements of section 520(f) of the act and this part and that the devices manufactured at that facility are adulterated under section 501(h) of the act.*

Basically, paragraph 21 CFR 820.1(d) requires foreign manufacturers to allow a full FDA inspection of their facilities as a condition of having their devices imported into the U.S. The inspection will be made against these CGMP regulations, and full compliance will be expected. If the foreign manufacturer refuses to permit an FDA inspection of the plant, FDA may declare the product to be adulterated and prevent its importation into the United States.

21 CFR 820.1(e) Exemptions or Variances. *(1) Any person who wishes to petition for an exemption or variance from any device quality system requirement is subject to the requirements of section 520(f)(2) of the act. Petitions for an exemption or variance shall be submitted according to the procedures set forth in § 10.30 of this chapter, the Food and Drug Administration's administrative procedures. Guidance is available from the Center for Devices and Radiological Health, Division of Small Manufacturers Assistance, Regulatory Assistance Branch (HFZ-220), 1350 Piccard Drive, Rockville, MD 20850 U.S.A., telephone 1-800-638-2041, or 1-301-443-6597, FAX 301-443-8818.*

(2) FDA may initiate and grant a variance from any device quality system requirement where the agency determines that such vari-

ance is in the best interest of the public health. Such variance will remain in effect only so long as there remains a public need for the device and the device would not likely be made sufficiently available without the variance.

Paragraph 21 CFR 820.1(e) is a notice that allows for exemptions or variances to the CGMP. The request for an exemption or variance may be initiated by a firm or the FDA itself. The paragraph is helpful in that provisions are made for useful exemptions or variances. In general these exemptions or variances are not all inclusive in nature. In other words, it is not likely that a blanket exemption from all parts of the CGMP will be granted. Only the most unreasonable or most costly requirements are granted exemptions, and there will be an expectation that where possible, CGMPs will be followed. In fact even if an exception or variance is granted, the manufacturer must still be able to provide assurance that the resulting devices will be safe and efficacious. These exemptions or variances are primarily useful for devices that are made in very small quantities or are custom made for a particular patient. In these cases there are often insufficient economies of scale, and the application of full CGMPs could cause the cost of the devices to become unreasonable.

The FDA has noted that until an exemption or variance is granted, the manufacturer should not deviate from the CGMP. Also, in the Quality System Manual, it was noted that designating the device as a "customized" device does not, by itself, exempt the device from CGMP requirements.

21 CFR 820.3 Definitions

Part 21 CFR 820.3 will be handled in a different manner from the other parts, because the definitions themselves do not require the preparation of separate documents. Where useful, the definition has been placed with the part in which the definition finds application, and this will be noted in place of the definition in this list. Definitions with general utility have not been placed with particular parts and are given here. It is important to know these definitions, because they may be different from what the reader may regard as the commonly accepted definitions.

21 CFR 820.3(a) Act *means the Federal Food, Drug, and Cosmetic Act as amended (secs. 201-903, 52 Stat. 1040 et seq., as amended*

(21 U.S.C. 321-394)). All definitions in section 201 of the act shall apply to these regulations.

21 CFR 820.3(b) Complaint; see 21 CFR 820.198.

21 CFR 820.3(c) Component *means any raw material, substance, piece, part, software, firmware, labeling, or assembly which is intended to be included as part of the finished, packaged, and labeled device.*

Note that components that are accessories for a device are often considered to be devices in their own right and may need to be treated like finished products.

21 CFR 820.3(d) Control number; see 21 CFR 820.162(e).

21 CFR 820.3(e) Design History File; see 21 CFR 820.30(j).

21 CFR 820.3(f) Design input; see 21 CFR 820.30(c).

21 CFR 820.3(g) Design output; see 21 CFR 820.30(d).

21 CFR 820.3(h) Design review; see 21 CFR 820.30(e).

21 CFR 820.3(i) Device history record; see 21 CFR 820.184.

21 CFR 820.3(j) Device master record; see 21 CFR 820.181.

21 CFR 820.3(k) Establish *means define, document (written or electronic), and implement.*

21 CFR 820.3(l) Finished Device *means any device or accessory to any device that is suitable for use or capable of functioning, whether or not it is packaged, labeled, or sterilized.*

21 CFR 820.3(m) Lot or batch *means one or more components or finished devices that consist of a single type, model, class, size, composition, and software version that are manufactured under essentially the same conditions and that are intended to have uniform characteristics and quality within specified limits.*

21 CFR 820.3(n) Management with executive responsibility; see 21 CFR 820.20.

21 CFR 820.3(o) Manufacturer *means any person who designs, manufactures, fabricates, assembles, or processes a finished device. Manufacturer includes but is not limited to those who perform the functions of contract sterilization, installation, relabeling, remanufacturing, repacking, or specification development, and initial distributors of foreign entities performing these functions.*

21 CFR 820.3(p) Manufacturing material; see 21 CFR 820.70(h).

21 CFR 820.3(q) Nonconformity; see 21 CFR 820.90(a).

21 CFR 820.3(r) Product *means components, manufacturing materials, in-process devices, finished devices, and returned devices.*

21 CFR 820.3(s) Quality *means the totality of features and characteristics that bear on the ability of a device to satisfy fitness-for-use, including safety and performance.*

21 CFR 820.3(t) Quality audit; see 21 CFR 820.22.

21 CFR 820.3(u) Quality policy; see 21 CFR 820.20.

21 CFR 820.3(v) Quality system; see 21 CFR 820.5.

21 CFR 820.3(w) Remanufacturer *means any person who processes, conditions, renovates, repackages, restores, or does any other act to a finished device that significantly changes the finished device's performance or safety specifications, or intended use.*

21 CFR 820.3(x) Rework; see 21 CFR 820.90(b)(2).

21 CFR 820.3(y) Specification *means any requirement with which a product, process, service, or other activity must conform.*

21 CFR 820.3(z) Validation; see 21 CFR 820.30 (g) and 21 CFR 820.75(a).

21 CFR 820.3(aa) Verification; see 21 CFR 820.30(f).

Part; This term is not really defined in any section, but it is used specifically to refer to 21 CFR 820 in its entirety, as in *this part,* when written into a regulation. The reader should be aware of this and realize that this usage is quite different from the usual definition of *part.* Also, beware of confusion with *part* as a component.

21 CFR 820.5 Quality System

Each manufacturer shall establish and maintain a quality system that is appropriate to the specific medical device(s) designed or manufactured, and that meets the requirements of this part.

21 CFR 820.3(v) Quality system *means the organizational structure, responsibilities, procedures, processes, and resources for implementing quality management.*

1. **Quality System Description.** Because establishing and maintaining quality system procedures and instructions is what the rest of the CGMP is all about, the Quality System document can be relatively simple. As will be seen when reviewing the rest of the regulations, the quality system goes beyond the traditional areas of quality assurance and quality control. The regulation of quality systems is based on the idea that the safety and efficacy of devices can be ensured by the development, implementation, and maintenance of procedures designed to execute specific requirements.

Departments and groups, such as Sales and Purchasing, that are not traditionally viewed as being a part of the quality organization must be included in the operations of the quality system. The document prepared for 21 CFR 820.5 should contain a description of the manufacturer's quality system. This could be a simple listing of quality system functions listed with their attendant responsibilities, that is, who is responsible for doing them and what are they responsible for doing? A type of organization chart could also be used with functions and responsibilities noted. As for resources, a simple statement that the manufacturer will provide the resources needed for the functioning of the quality system should suffice. As this document will be routed through the manufacturer's management for approval, this commitment will be documented. Note that if the definition is considered, the quality system is basically the organization needed for managing the quality activities that the manufacturer needs for producing a licensed product. It may not be necessary to have a Quality System Manager or department if there are appropriate activities being conducted within existing departments. In reality, it is often useful to have a small group that monitors and coordinates quality-related activities within the company. Certain departments such as Purchasing or Sales may have only a small involvement with the quality system, and it is useful to have people who can work with these departments to ensure that quality activities are conducted when necessary. It is important to remember that, if a unit performs a quality system function, it will, to the extent of the function, be expected to meet quality system requirements.

※ Subpart B—Quality System ※ Requirements

21 CFR 820.20 Management Responsibility

21 CFR 820.20(a) Quality Policy. Management with executive responsibility shall establish its policy and objectives for, and commitment to, quality. Management with executive responsibility *shall ensure that the quality policy is understood, implemented, and maintained at all levels of the organization.*

21 CFR 820.3(n) Management with executive responsibility *means those senior employees of a manufacturer who have the authority to establish or make changes to the manufacturer's quality policy and quality system.*

21 CFR 820.3(u) Quality policy *means the overall quality intentions and direction of an organization with respect to quality, as established by management with executive responsibility.*

2. **Quality Policy.** The Quality Policy is usually a brief paragraph in which the upper management of the company states the company's commitment to quality and the quality goals that the company will strive to attain. This policy is often framed and posted in places such as reception areas, employee bulletin boards, and even on the backs of business cards. The problem that develops is in the second part of the regulation. There is a similar requirement in the ANSI/ISO/ASQC 9000 set of standards, and most ISO auditors know that companies are often deficient in disseminating their quality policy to all levels of the organization. If an auditor is looking for citations, one may usually be generated by finding an employee who is low in the hierarchy and discussing the company's quality policy with that individual. It really does a company little good to have upper management issue a quality policy with pious comments about it being "job number one" and then proceed to create conditions that prevent employees from having the policy as an attainable goal. All that this produces is cynicism in the workplace.

   The Quality Policy document should instruct management on the creation and maintenance of a company quality policy. It should describe how the employees (especially new hires) will be informed about the policy and what training will be done to ensure that the employees will understand the implications of the policy. This training may need to be periodically repeated, as company growth and development will usually result in a need for changes in the quality policy. Some companies have been known to prepare pamphlets that are given to employees to serve as references when the employees seek guidance on quality issues.

21 CFR 820.20(b) Organization. *Each manufacturer shall establish and maintain an adequate organizational structure to ensure that devices are produced in accordance with the requirements of this part.*

(1) Responsibility and authority. *Each manufacturer shall establish the appropriate responsibility, authority, and interrelation of all personnel who manage, perform, and verify work affecting quality, and provide the independence and authority necessary to perform these tasks.*

(2) Resources. *Each manufacturer shall provide adequate resources, including the assignment of trained personnel, for management, performance of work, and verification activities, including internal quality audits, to carry out the requirements of this part.*

(3) Management representative. *Management with executive responsibility shall appoint, and document such appointment of a member of management who, irrespective of other responsibilities, shall have established authority over and responsibility for:*

> **(i)** *Ensuring that quality system requirements are effectively established and effectively maintained in accordance with this part; and*

> **(ii)** *Reporting on the performance of the quality system to management with executive responsibility for review.*

3. **Quality System Organization.** The first thing needed to fulfill the requirements of 21 CFR 820.20(b) is an organization chart of the manufacturer's quality system. This organization chart should show that the workers in the quality system are independent enough to avoid conflicts of interest when performing their duties. The workers' responsibilities and authority should be written into their position descriptions or work assignments. FDA has stated that the manufacturer must assign the responsibility and authority and provide organizational freedom or independence to employees who initiate action to prevent nonconformities; identify and document quality problems; initiate, recommend, provide, and verify solutions to quality problems; and direct or control further processing, delivery, or installation of nonconforming product. The actual document written to satisfy these organization requirements should require the preparation and maintenance of the organization chart and state the responsibility and authority that must be granted to each of the positions. A review of this document should provide the reviewer

with a clear conclusion that the manufacturer has made a commitment to have a functional quality system. The requirement for an "adequate organizational structure" is fairly flexible and will be interpreted by inspectors in the light of the complexity of the company and the device being manufactured, as well as its potential for injuring an operator or patient. In general, members of the quality organization, including those who are responsible for quality control, should not report directly to a manager responsible for manufacturing operations.

While this reporting structure is not specifically prohibited by the regulations, it poses a clear potential for conflicts of interest. Companies that create these structures should be prepared to explain their reasoning for the reporting relationship and also for the method by which the organizational freedom or independence of the quality organization is maintained. An auditor or inspector will frequently encounter organizations that have tried their best to suppress quality activities by keeping the quality organization at a low level, always reporting to a person with little or no knowledge of the field of Quality.

A frequently encountered mistake occurs when the company believes that the only reason for engaging in quality activities is to meet regulatory requirements. In reality, a quality system should produce a considerable amount of information that will be useful in the management of the company and its processes. Information on the quality of purchased goods, numbers of deviation notices, and failure of distributed products should be factored into the thinking of the company's management. When a company is only trying to meet regulatory requirements, it will tend to ignore these data and may even avoid collecting useful information.

Subparagraph (2) does not require a separate document of its own. It is mainly a regulation to prevent the manufacturer from denying resources to its quality system. A claim that the quality system was unable to function due to lack of resources will usually be met with a statement that this is a cost of doing business, and if one is in business, one had better be prepared to provide resources to all vital operations, including quality.

Subparagraph (3) basically calls for the appointment of a manager of quality systems who will have the authority and responsibility for the two activities mentioned in that subparagraph. These requirements should be written into the position description or work assignment for the position. If this position is not a separate position in its own right, the assignment of the authority and responsibility to a particular position should be documented. Regardless of the organizational structure, responsibility without authority creates a bad situation. This problem can easily arise when a manager is given the responsibility, but is easily and frequently overruled by higher level managers for reasons of convenience or politics.

21 CFR 820.20(c) Management Review. *Management with executive responsibility shall review the suitability and effectiveness of the quality system at defined intervals and at sufficient frequency according to established procedures to ensure that the quality system satisfies the requirements of this part and the manufacturer's established quality policy and objectives. The results of quality system reviews shall be documented.*

4. **Quality System Review.** This document needs to establish a quality systems review committee. The composition of the committee will vary with the manufacturer's organizational type, but at a minimum, should include the supervisor of the manager designated in 21 CFR 820.20(b)(3) and the individual responsible for providing resources for the quality system. The frequency of committee meetings should be given. The frequency of these meetings will depend upon the complexity of the manufacturer's quality system and the number of quality problems confronting the committee. At a minimum, the meetings should be frequent enough to ensure that all parts of the quality system receive adequate review. If the manager designated in 21 CFR 820.20(b)(3) is already monitoring the performance of the quality system, the meetings could be bimonthly or quarterly. The Quality System Review document should also specify the key items to be reviewed, including items such as summaries of internal quality audits, defect or reject rates, and customer complaints. Subjects to be reviewed could include: the organizational structure, adequacy of resources including staffing, failure rates, and purchaser or internal comments about the device. Basically, the information to be reviewed should be indicative of

the proper functioning of the quality system and should include some basic statistical descriptors, such as Pareto charts and trend analysis. The internal quality auditing program (see 21 CFR 820.22) should serve as one basic source of information for this activity. The idea is to show that the quality policies and objectives are being met and that the quality system continues to be suitable and effective. This management review should be a broad-based review in contrast to the unit-specific focus of quality audits.

The management review and any recommendations or actions resulting from the review must be reported in a document that will become a part of the quality system records (21 CFR 820.186). This report is a protected document under the provisions of 21 CFR 820.180(c) and does not have to be given to or copied for FDA employees. Therefore, the document should be candid in dealing with any problems of the quality system. Upon request from the FDA, the chair of the review committee may need to prepare, date, and sign a document certifying that the reviews did take place and that the requirements of 21 CFR 820.180(c) were met.

21 CFR 820.20(d) Quality Planning. *Each manufacturer shall establish a quality plan which defines the quality practices, resources, and activities relevant to devices that are designed and manufactured. The manufacturer shall establish how the requirements for quality will be met.*

5. **Quality Planning.** The Quality Planning document is a general document that describes the manufacturer's plans for implementing its quality system in general. Specific quality planning for a specific device should be addressed as part of the design process covered by 21 CFR 820.30, but the overall planning that deals with areas not covered by the design process should be described in this document. The Quality Planning document should contain a description of the manufacturer's plans for implementing CGMP requirements, the structure and interrelationships among personnel and functions with responsibilities for quality, and a discussion of short- and long-range goals for the company's quality system. Also of interest will be descriptions of the interfaces between the quality functions and other departments.

21CFR 820.20(e) Quality System Procedures. *Each manufacturer shall establish quality system procedures and instructions. An outline of the structure of the documentation used in the quality system shall be established where appropriate.*

6. **Quality System Outline.** The procedures that are to be implemented in 21 CFR 820.20(d) need to be written and entered into the documentation system. The quality system, itself, needs to be described and documented. The documentation should include procedural documents as well as policies. An organization chart of the documentation system needs to be described. The outline of the structure of the documentation system does not need to include every document that the manufacturer has, but it should include documents that are related to the operation of the quality system and the manufacturing of the device. The outline (or organization chart) could be built using document groups and those documents that stand alone. In a separate section, such as in footnotes to the chart, the groups could be shown with the individual documents that belong to the groups listed with the individual group.

This outline of the quality system documents is the same as that which will be found in section 4.2.1 of ANSI/ISO/ASQC 9001:1994. The difference is that FDA only requires that it be prepared when appropriate. Manufacturers with simple quality systems may not need to meet this requirement. If the outline is prepared, the manufacturer should also review the ISO requirement if it wishes to be in compliance with ANSI/ISO/ASQC 9001:1994 as well.

21 CFR 820.22 Quality Audit

Each manufacturer shall establish procedures for quality audits and conduct such audits to assure that the quality system is in compliance with the established quality system requirements and to determine the effectiveness of the quality system. Quality audits shall be conducted by individuals who do not have direct responsibility for the matters being audited. Corrective action(s), including a reaudit of deficient matters, shall be taken when necessary. A report of the results of each quality audit, and reaudit(s) where taken, shall be made and such reports shall be reviewed by management having responsibility for the matters audited. The dates and results of quality audits and reaudits shall be documented.

21 CFR 820.3(t) Quality audit *means an established systematic, independent, examination of a manufacturer's quality system that is performed at defined intervals and at sufficient frequency to ensure that both quality system activities and the results of such activities comply with specified quality system procedures, that these procedures are implemented effectively, and that these procedures are suitable to achieve quality system objectives.*

Several documents are required to fulfill the requirements of 21 CFR 820.22. They include documents covering Internal Audits, External Audits, Audit Procedures and Standards, Audit Reports, and Audit Reviews; and are explained in detail as follows.

7. **Internal Audit Policies.** The first document needed in the quality records is a policy document that establishes the requirement for internal quality audits, their frequency, and their purpose as stated in the regulation. The departments or administrative units that are to be audited should be noted and the standards, company policies, ISO, EN, CGMP, and so on against which they will be assessed should be specified. The audits should not only address the issue of whether or not units are following the proper procedures and instructions, but also whether or not the procedures and instructions themselves are adequate for CGMP purposes and for manufacturing a product that will meet quality requirements. All units, including the administrative offices and the auditing function itself, must be audited, but not all units require the same audit frequency. The importance and difficulty of the activity that a unit is responsible for performing should be reflected in the audit frequency. For instance, Purchasing may be audited on an annual basis, while a manufacturing department that produces a complex subunit may need to be audited quarterly. This document should also require the inspection of equipment maintenance schedules as part of an internal audit (21 CFR 820.70(g)(2)).

These audits are of the type known as *first party* or internal audits. In other words, the company audits itself to check on the proper functioning of its quality system. These audits should be announced and scheduled well in advance of the actual audit date. All company functions should be subject to some level of auditing. The receptionist at the front desk can have a high impact on the way that a company is perceived by an auditor, inspector, or visiting customer; while the janitor who combines radioactive waste with normal trash may be exposing the company to more than just radiation. Auditor independence is an important issue and is a key factor in assessing the quality of the audit itself. If necessary a consultant could be hired to perform an audit of the auditing function. The general rule is that the auditors must not have responsibilities over the areas being audited.

The definition of "manufacturer" has been extended to cover contract sterilizers, specification developers, repackagers, relabelers and initial distributors because these individuals may have an impact upon the safety or efficacy of the device. Consequently, to the extent that the manufacturer has control over these individuals, they should be subject to auditing, as they may be regarded to be an integral part of the manufacturing process.

8. **External Audit Policies.** In the event that the company engages in external or second party auditing as a part of its vendor control (see 21 CFR 820.50), a second policy document should be written to cover this class of audits. These audits are essentially the same as internal audits, except that the vendor's whole quality system is potentially subject to the audit and all departments may be audited on a given day. However, because of time constraints, particular departments or processes may be targeted in a particular audit. The targeting should arise from the concerns of the manufacturer, especially if there is a history of quality problems or if there is a concern about a particular weakness in a component. External audits of suppliers or contractors may be needed to verify that suppliers or contractors are following appropriate CGMP rules. This procedure may become especially important in situations where testing or inspection of the incoming material cannot ensure its safety or efficacy, or where a vendor is CGMP compliant only because of contractual requirements. Changes in the quality of the product supplied may trigger a need for an audit, especially if there is an indication that the level of unit to unit variation has increased. Similarly, changes in a company's management or high personnel turnover may indicate a need for a review of the vendor's commitment to quality practices.

Foreign suppliers or vendors, in particular, may need to be audited. Problems arising from geographic or cultural separation may need to be addressed along with the usual compliance with the CGMP regulations. Note that there are some countries that have their own GMP regulations. These countries may also certify their companies to be GMP compliant. In turn, these companies may seek to avoid an audit by stating that they are GMP compliant and are certified by their national body. The problem here is that until an audit is performed to verify this status, these are just claims. In particular, the company may be compliant with its country's GMP's, but these might be quite different from U.S. CGMP's, or the compliance may be lax. The manufacturer is responsible for showing that its supplier can meet U.S. standards, and this responsibility cannot be shed by simply referring to foreign certificates of compliance.

As with internal audits, external audits should be preannounced and scheduled with the auditee. Auditors should resist the development of a police mentality. The fact is that the auditor has no judicial authority, except for those spelled out in contracts, and should be careful not to offend the auditee as good audits require a cooperative attitude on the part of the auditor and auditee.

9. **Auditing Procedures and Standards.** This document should establish the procedures to be followed in auditing and the qualification requirements for auditors. Although FDA removed the requirement that auditors should be "appropriately trained" from 21 CFR 820.22, the requirement still exists as a part of 21 CFR 820.25 which requires all employees to be appropriately trained. Auditors should be trained, especially if external audits are to be conducted. It is critical that auditors follow basic ethical and procedural standards to minimize conflict and lack of cooperation. The use of American Society for Quality (ASQ) or Registrar Accreditation Board (RAB) certified auditors, at least as the lead, or supervising, auditors is recommended. Certification of RAB or ASQ training should be a part of the auditor's training records (see 21 CFR 820.25(b)). Some larger companies also have internal training programs for auditors as they realize that the actions of auditors are crucial to the quality of their quality programs.

The standards against which the audits will be conducted must be specified. The parts of the Code of Federal Regulations, the EN or ISO standard, internal operation documents, or contract specifications must be stated for internal as well as external audits. In cases where an external audit is being conducted on a supplier, the auditors will need to be aware of the information developed in response to 21 CFR 820.50 and any contractual arrangements between the companies. Contracts exist where the supplier is not required to meet CGMP standards in general or where certain CGMP sections or paragraphs are excluded from consideration. These types of contracts are often the result of having a Purchasing department that is unsophisticated in the ways of GMP. Therefore, companies must be vigilant in looking out for their own interests and assume that others are doing the same.

Well-trained auditors are very important. During an external audit, they act as representatives of the manufacturer's quality system before the manufacturer's vendors. During internal audits, the auditors act as representatives of upper management in assessing the operations of the quality system. It is crucial that these auditors have good people skills, as well as being well versed in the standards that will be used for the audit. Auditors with bad manners and interrogation techniques that make them appear to have been trained by the Gestapo or KGB will alienate employees or degrade the manufacturer's reputation. Auditors who are ignorant of manufacturing or technical realities will look like fools and further damage the manufacturer's or the quality system department's image to the point where the auditees will develop a contemptuous attitude. Future audits will be met with hostility and non-cooperation. In addition, some auditees are extremely paranoid in their defensiveness. An untrained or poorly trained auditor will almost certainly fail in dealing with these individuals, and this will degrade the quality of the audit. Among trained auditors, it is taken as a basic principle that the greatest benefit from the audit will be derived by the auditee. This principle must be kept in mind if a manufacturer wishes to have a successful auditing program.

10. **Audit Reports.** Another document should address the procedures and format for the audit reports, corrective action request (CAR) forms, and audit closure certificates. Procedural docu-

ments for audits should define who is being audited, what is being audited, against what standards is the audit being conducted, what are the special considerations for the audit, the frequency and specific date of the audit. Another part of the document should describe how the audits are to be conducted. Will checklists be used or will it be purely verbal, what reports will be generated, who will receive and review them, and when will the final report be issued? The format of corrective action requests and audit closure certificates should be described.

Corrective action requests often arise from deficiencies found during an audit, and audit closure certificates are issued when the auditee has completed all actions required in the audit report. This document should specify a system of document control numbers for assignment to each audit and corresponding audit report. This will aid in collecting all documents related to a particular audit and in cross-referencing among audit reports, especially if an electronic documentation system is being employed. A file location or designation should be established to contain audit reports and their associated paperwork. The names and responsibilities of all auditors should be preserved in the audit reports. Training classes will provide auditing and report models that could be incorporated into company procedures. These activities should be closely coordinated with those in 21 CFR 820.20(d), 21 CFR 820.40 and 21 CFR 820.186. Remember that these reports are protected documents under the provisions of 21 CFR 820.180(c), and this means that they must be separated from other documents that may be reviewed or copied by FDA personnel. The protection afforded by 21 CFR 820.180(c) does not cover the audit procedural documents, corrective action requests and reports, and the management reviews of audits. These documents may be reviewed by FDA personnel and they should be prepared with that possibility in mind.

11. **Audit Reviews.** Responsibilities and review requirements, especially management review, should be established and documentation procedures established for the review, follow-up, and closure of CARs and the audit in general. This should also address the conditions for initiating reaudits. Reaudits should be scheduled on a regular basis and may vary in frequency, depending on the level of concern over the operations of a department or

supplier. A deterioration in the quality of output or supplies or a failure to comply with CARs within the time frame specified should trigger reviews to determine if a reaudit is warranted. The nature of the reviews and the personnel to be involved should be specified. These activities should be coordinated with the management review of 21 CFR 820.20(c) and the corrective actions in 21 CFR 820.100.

In particular, this document should specify the format of the audit review. In many companies there is sort of an "audit, file, and forget" system which basically arises from an attitude that addresses the form (We need to audit, so we'll do it.) but not the spirit (What does the audit tells us?) of the regulation. For the audit to be valuable, management needs to review the audit report with the auditor, and pay particular attention to the responses received from the auditee. Remember that an audit is not complete until the auditee has had an opportunity to respond to the findings and clear up any misunderstandings that may have arisen. The audit review, therefore, should not be performed until the auditee has had an opportunity to respond to a draft audit report. This audit review can occur as a review of a specific audit report or a periodic review of all reports generated over a certain interval. It is during this meeting that a management evaluation of the auditee should be performed.

Some organizations employ what is called "continuous auditing." This practice should be avoided. At the very least it implies a lack of confidence in the supervisory employees in the area subject to the continuous auditing. At worst, it can degenerate into supervisory control by the auditors, who are unlikely to have the expertise required for running the particular department. During their training auditors are instructed not to propose solutions to problems that they encounter. Some auditors disregard these instructions and go about spouting information and solutions. The problem is that the auditee, not the auditor, should be the expert in the particular area. Quite often an auditee will deliberately allow an auditor to make an erroneous suggestion and then, later, come up with the statement that "we were only doing what the auditor said." Even worse situations can develop, and the auditor who allows ego to take over thinking will create many problems.

21 CFR 820.25 Personnel

21 CFR 820.25(a) General.   Each manufacturer shall employ suffi-cient personnel with the necessary education, background, training, and experience to ensure that all activities required by this part are correctly performed.

Although a separate document may not be required for this gen-eral requirement, its provisions should be incorporated into many other documents such as hiring policies and position descriptions. Auditors should also be aware of the requirements of parts (a) and (b) here as the consequences are far reaching. Basically, the require-ment states that there shall be sufficient numbers of capable em-ployees available to perform the work required to meet the require-ments of 21 CFR 820. Therefore a claim that the manufacturer was unable to comply with a provision of the Quality System regulations because of a lack of personnel or facilities or of trained personnel immediately places the manufacturer in violation of this section.

21 CFR 820.25(b) Training.   Each manufacturer shall establish pro-cedures for identifying training needs and ensure that all personnel are trained to adequately perform their assigned responsibilities. Training shall be documented.

(1) As part of their training, personnel shall be made aware of de-vice defects which may occur from the improper performance of their specific jobs.

(2) Personnel who perform verification and validation activities shall be made aware of defects and errors that may be encountered as part of their job functions.

12. **Training Requirements.** This document should specify general training requirements for the company and specify that depart-ments should ensure adequate training of their personnel and document that training. All employees should receive training, from qualified individuals, that is appropriate to their function in the company. This training should be specific to the needs of the particular job. General employee training may be done with new employees, but each employee should also be trained in the special requirements for the particular job. Also all em-ployees should be trained in the requirements of the quality sys-tem so that a general awareness of quality requirements will

exist within the company. It is a basic tenet of quality management that all units of a company participate in the manufacturing of a device, and the manufacturing is the result of an integrated activity involving all units. Many companies perform the first, general training on CGMP and general quality matters as a part of the new employee orientation program. A form for recording internal and external training should be developed. Training should be continuous. Not only do the CGMPs evolve over time, but also guidelines change, as do standard methods for dealing with the CGMPs. Provision should be made for the annual training of employees on recent developments in coping with the CGMPs. In addition to this, employees should be trained to perform their jobs. Periodic training to maintain skills is important, as technology changes and skills that are infrequently used are forgotten. Also, it is important to teach employees about the defects that they may encounter and instruct them about the consequences that may result if they should fail to perform their jobs properly. Managers and supervisors must keep up to date on current theories and methods for management as well as quality. Provisions should also be made for safety, first aid, hazardous material, disaster response, human resources, and other training related to the working environment.

The regulation makes the statement that personnel shall be "trained to adequately perform" their duties. This carries with it the implication that the training must be effective, and a mechanism must exist by which the company verifies the efficacy of a training program. It is not sufficient to place an employee in a training class and simply verify the employee's physical presence during the training. Some company trainers and training consultants actually use examinations that are then placed in employee files to show that the material was learned. In other cases, supervisors of a work area will issue a certificate verifying the efficacy of the training based upon observation of the employee's work. Employers should also take advantage of the many societies, such as the ASQ, that provide training and certification programs where the employee is examined to verify training and subjected to periodic renewal or upgrading requirements.

It is important to have the whole company functioning as an integrated quality system, and this can only be established through training that ensures that each employee, including the CEO and Vice Presidents, will understand their role in the quality system. It is management's responsibility to define the content of the activities that should be directed at training each employee to perform assigned functions.

In the original form of the proposed GMPs there were several sections that explicitly stated that certain actions were to be performed by "qualified" or "trained" individuals. In many cases, these statements were removed in favor of 21 CFR 820.25(a) and (b) as these regulations basically state that employees must be qualified to do their jobs correctly. These requirements apply to all employees including temporaries and consultants. Based on this rule, it is assumed that if the manufacturer used an employee for a certain function, the employee was qualified to perform the function.

13. **Training Files.** The location and contents of training files should be specified. Each employee's training and experience should be documented, including brief summaries of preemployment reference checks that were aimed at determining the employee's experience relative to the job being filled. Because of their confidential nature, personal data should not be inserted in training files. The training files should be distinct from personnel files. In most companies, training files for active employees are held by departments or groups, and when the employee leaves employment, the file is transferred to the Personnel (Human Resources) department for long-term maintenance. With an electronic document system, the training files could be held in a single memory device, separate from the one that holds personnel records, that is protected from unauthorized access. Where necessary, specific training, certification, or qualification requirements should be written into position descriptions and a record made of the satisfaction of the requirements. This can be especially useful for temporary employees and consultants. Since they are usually with the company for a short period, their previous experience and qualifications should be on file to show that they were capable of performing their jobs correctly.

Note that 21 CFR 820.25(a) refers to the education, background, and experience of the employee in addition to the employee's training. Many regulations state that employees must be qualified by reason of "training and experience." For these reasons the training files should contain information on an employee's education and prior experience in addition to the training provided by the company. Information on education and prior experience provided by a candidate for employment should be spot checked, verified, and documented. Remember that the mere possession of a degree in a certain area may not qualify an employee to perform a particular function such as design control or complaint handling. Specific training will be needed.

※ Subpart C—Design Controls ※

21 CFR 820.30 Design Controls

This section on design controls contains much of what is new in these revised GMP regulations. Those companies that are already complying with the requirements of EN 46001 and ANSI/ISO/ASQC 9001 should already have much of this in place. Those that are not yet meeting EN 46001 and ANSI/ISO/ASQC 9001 standards should plan their work on design controls to meet ISO standards as well as GMP needs. The differences, really, are small and will be covered later in this book. The regulations covering design controls should be viewed as providing a quality assurance system for the design of a particular product.

The FDA has recognized the confusion and concern that has developed over the introduction of requirements for design controls into the CGMP. Consequently, CDRH has issued and plans to issue several guidelines, three of which are mentioned in this book, to aid workers new to the field. They also provided an additional year for manufacturers to come into compliance with the design control regulations. Consequently, although the new CGMP as given in 21 CFR 820 became effective on June 1, 1997, compliance with the design control requirements as covered in 21 CFR 820.30 will not be required until June 1, 1998. During the additional year, FDA will expect manufacturers to make reasonable efforts to comply with the regulations of 21 CFR 820.30 but will not expect full compliance.

The requirements for design control will not be applied retroactively, but on June 1, 1997, they will apply to designs that are in the development phase and a design and development plan should be in place. Full compliance will be expected on June 1, 1998. When changes are made to new or existing designs after June 1, 1997, the application of design controls will be expected. Basically, the FDA has said that while they will expect compliance beginning in June of 1997, they will not issue citations for noncompliance until June 1998.

A major question that will arise is, "When, during product development, do we need to comply with design control requirements?" Similar questions often arise in the areas of drugs and biologics during the transition from R & D to GLP (21 CFR 58) and GMP (21 CFR 210, 211) regulated activities. The usual answer is something like, "You need to start complying when you reach the point where you know that you are going to try to develop a product." The problem here, of course, is that a device company usually does not know that it is going to try to develop a product until after a feasibility study has been completed. This feasibility study needs to be based on a particular design. The results of a feasibility study are only useful within the context of a specific design, and the development of that design should have taken place under design control requirements. A suggested rule here might be that all designs must be developed under the provisions of 21 CFR 820.30. It is disingenuous to have a large R & D program and later claim that 90 percent of its output had nothing to do with the development of the device that is about to be manufactured.

This requirement may lead to some conflict with R & D personnel because there will be an undefined, diffuse point when R & D sketches, proposals, and concepts turn into the preliminary design that will eventually be tested in a feasibility study. The best approach here is to require the R & D function to meet design control requirements for the preparation of all design proposals that are submitted for feasibility studies and to prepare a clear summary of events involved in the development of the proposed design. The company should look upon this transition as that point where R & D concepts change into executable designs.

The Food and Drug Administration, in the form of CDRH, realized that the introduction of design control requirements into the device CGMPs would create problems for manufacturers who have not previously been required to comply with these elements. Consequently, in March 1996, CDRH issued for review and comment, two guidance documents to help to provide manufacturers with information on the factors that must be considered when planning compliance activities. One document entitled, "Do It By Design: An Introduction to Human Factors in Medical Devices," is exactly that; a primer for those who are unfamiliar with human factors engineering. The second document was entitled, "Design Control Guidance for Medical Device Manufacturers," and it is provided as a guidance document for compliance with 21 CFR 820.30 and Subclause 4.4 of ANSI/ISO/ASQC 9001. Both of these documents are fairly well written and should be obtained by manufacturers who will need to develop procedures for activities related to design controls. The documents are available from CDRH as printed copies or via their fax or Internet systems.

Both of these documents and the Quality System Manual were used to develop the following discussion of the requirements of 21 CFR 820.30. Where there were specific or brief statements applicable to what follows, a specific quotation or direction is given. However, if the discussion is more general, reference to "Do It By Design" or to the "Design Control Guidance" or the "Quality System Manual" will be made.

There is some controversy over the guidance documents. CDRH has repeatedly stated that guidelines are not regulations and are geared to help the novice, but guidelines have often been used as minimum standards for enforcement, and many manufacturers are wary of them. The point here is that, if a manufacturer wishes to deviate or depart from a guideline, it is the manufacturer's responsibility to show that the procedure finally adopted is at least equivalent to the one given in the guideline. The evidence for this equivalence is often lacking.

The guidelines, in addition to providing specific instructions for parts of 21 CFR 820.30, also describe a general structure for the project team. While there is no explicit statement requiring the use of this team structure, the description of responsibilities and requirements for independence of function will lead the reader to conclude that the requirements of 21 CFR 820.30 could be best met with that organization. All members of the project team should be technically competent at least to the point of being able to understand their role and function in the project. Basically, the project team needs to contain several subunits or functions that will act independently but also in a coordinated manner. This structure will accommodate the multiple cycles of design, development, and review that will take place as a device proceeds from concept to finished product. It is important that all major functional units that will be involved with the project be represented on the team. Thus there should be representatives from manufacturing, marketing, engineering, quality systems, R & D, and purchasing who are directly involved as members of various subunits of the team. These individuals should have full authority to act as representatives of their units. Nothing impedes progress more than having team members who constantly need to check with their supervisors before being able to make or accept a decision. If a supervisor is that concerned with the decisions of the team, the supervisor should become a member and replace the subordinate.

The project team should have an administrative subteam that will have executive responsibility and will be in communication with upper management. This group will be responsible for training issues such as the need for training in risk management and human factors engineering. It would be responsible for identifying structural barriers that impede the progress of the project and for coordinating the activities of the team with groups that are not directly represented on the project team. This group will be described in more detail under 21 CFR 820.30(a).

A design development team would have the responsibility of actually developing the design and, finally, working with manufacturing to initiate the production of the finished device. This group should contain the individuals who developed the original device concept and proved its feasibility, but should not be limited to them as the manufacture and distribution of a device will require talents other than those of the developers. It will be responsible for the design inputs and outputs. Even after the device is in full production, this group will need to remain in existence to handle the evolution of the device as technology changes and manufacturing and marketing feedback are obtained. This group will be described in more detail under 21 CFR 820.30(c).

The design review group will have the responsibility for all design reviews, verifications, and validations. It will also be responsible for configuration control and document continuity. Paragraph, 21 CFR 820.30(e), specifically states that one or more individuals who do not have direct responsibility for design development shall be assigned by management to participate in design reviews. It would seem wise to place one of these individuals at the head of the design review group, and also to set a policy that no member of the design review group shall be subordinate to anyone in the design development team. The design review group will need to have sufficient authority to initiate the reviews and control changes as will be described in 21 CFR 820.30(e). As with the design development team, this group will need to remain in existence even after a product is being distributed. Design changes during a device's lifetime will require reviews and validations.

The size and complexity of the company and the device will determine the size of these subteams. A large company with a complex product for treating a critically ill patient may have subteams of twenty or more individuals, and, if the subteams threaten to become too large, they may need to form more subteams than those described above. On the other hand, a small company with a simple device might have a project team composed of only three people with no need for subteams. Each manufacturer needs to assess its own needs and limitations within the context of the regulations and guidelines. The individuals in the project team must have responsibilities and accountabilities within the context of the team. Major problems can arise if team members are only accountable to supervisors in their functional groups and are not accountable for their performance as members of the project team.

21 CFR 820.30(j) Design History File. *Each manufacturer shall establish and maintain a DHF for each type of device. The DHF shall contain or reference all records necessary to demonstrate that the design was developed in accordance with the approved design plan and the requirements of this part.*

21 CFR 820.3(e) Design History File *means a compilation of records which describe the complete design history of a finished device.*

Note that 21 CFR 820.30(j) is being taken out of sequence. The documents that follow should all be a part of the Design History File (DHF) so the description of the file has been placed ahead of these sections.

14. **Design History File.** The first document necessary for 21 CFR 820.30(j) will be the one that establishes the Design History File. It should contain the following information:

a. A description of the Design History File (for instance, that it is a file of quality documents related to a certain device design) and names of the types of documents that it will contain.

   The DHF must describe the complete history of the design of a particular device or component assembly of a device. For instance, if a company uses a certain subassembly (like a computer or detector) in several devices, it may make sense to have a separate DHF for this unit. The DHF should cover the development of the device, accessories, major components, labeling, packaging, and the manufacturing process. Even though every step in the design phase of the device may not be documented, the whole design history should be apparent from the contents of the DHF. The DHF must reference or contain enough records to prove that the design was developed in accordance with a design and development plan and other regulatory and design control requirements of the CGMP. The final design output from the design phase should be present in the DHF either as filed documents or by reference. The documents in the DHF will serve as the basis for creating the Device Master Record (DMR), which is described in 21 CFR 820.181. Remember, if the firm has more than one device design under development, more than one DHF will need preparation. Each device family needs its own DHF. If it may be argued that similar devices are simple variants of a single familial design, then a single DHF may be warranted. Each distinct design type should have its own DHF.

b. The system (if any) for designating which documents will be a part of this file. The DHF should contain the design and development plan, results of design reviews, design validation and verification results, and any other data needed to show compliance with design requirements. The DHF should contain or reference all of the documents that will demonstrate compliance with the design plan and the CGMP. In other words, all documents required by 21 CFR 820.30. The design control procedures should also be included in the DHF. Older versions of the DMR should be archived in the DHF. A carefully prepared index of its contents will be especially important if the file does not physically exist, but is only a section in a database.

c. The location of the file (physical or electronic), the name of the department responsible for maintaining the file, and a designation of the individual (by position) responsible for entering information and documents into the file.

d. The DHF serves as a long-term memory for the company, so that successive generations of workers may understand the history of how the device was developed and what decisions were made and for what reason. It will contain the verification and validation studies and also the safety and failure mode studies that may be referenced in the event that problems develop. The file should be named for the design that it will contain and also be labeled with any product or design codes for the device. This is important if several code names or numerical designations are used for prototypes, design intermediates, and the final device. In some companies, the file number for the DHF will become the part number of the finished device so that the continuity of the numbering system can be used to trace documents and parts through their system. Cross-indexing and key words are important here.

21 CFR 820.30(a) General. **(1)** *Each manufacturer of any class III, or class II device, and the class I devices listed in paragraph (a)(2) of this section, shall establish and maintain procedures to control and verify the design of the device in order to ensure that specified design requirements are met.* **(2)** *The following class I devices are subject to design controls:*

(i) *Devices automated with computer software; and*
(ii) *The devices listed in the following chart.*

Section	*Device*
868.6810	*Catheter, Tracheobronchial Suction*
878.4460	*Glove, Surgeon's*
880.6760	*Restraint, Protective*
892.5650	*System, Applicator, Radionuclide, Manual*
892.5740	*Source, Radionuclide Teletherapy*

15. **General Design Control.** This section of the regulations defines the devices that are subject to design controls. The resulting Design Control document must describe the general procedures to control and verify the design of the device. The classification of the device and the rationale for it should be given. This document will tell how the product design will be developed, reviewed, and released to manufacturing. It should be a general document, as the following documents will cover the specifics of how the procedures are to be executed. As almost all designs will evolve as they proceed from concept to manufactured product, procedures will be needed to allow for the updating of designs and revision procedures for design execution. This document should become a part of the DHF.

The Guideline on Design Control assigns certain responsibilities to senior management. These are:

a. Decide on how and by whom the design process is to be managed. Presumably this would involve naming the team leader and determining the structure of the subteams.

b. Ensure that adequate resources are available to carry out the design process in the time required.

c. Ensure that internal policies are established to deal with issues affecting the design process. This would involve ensuring that functions such as manufacturing are integrated into the team to the degree necessary for the project.

d. Ensure that skills needed for the project are available, and that authorization is granted for training, hiring, or contracting for missing skills.

e. Ensure that equipment and other resources necessary for the development of the manufacturing process are available as the need develops.

In addition, the quality system manager with executive responsibility must work closely with the team management to identify and implement quality requirements for the project. This would include establishing quality policies that impact the design process. For large projects, a separate project quality plan may need to be developed.

The responsibilities of senior management must be expressed in this document. It should then go on to describe the formation of a product design team and give the responsibilities of the various subsections of the team. These would be the project manager and administrative team, the design group itself, and the design review group. Basically, the administrative team should be composed of the project manager (team leader) and representatives from major functional groups, including the heads of the subteams, whose participation will be important for the development and licensing of the device. These would be representatives of manufacturing, engineering, quality systems, regulatory affairs, and so on. Also, other departments may need to be periodically represented. For instance, when the raw material specifications are developed, it will be useful to have a representative of the purchasing department present. Sufficient staff should also be assigned to the project team to allow for planning activities, administering the budget, training the whole team, communicating and coordinating activities with upper management and departments that are not directly represented on the team, and providing general support for the project manager who would probably be a senior manager with a full-time responsibility for the development of the device.

The training that is required involves general training in the CGMP, human factors awareness, and risk management. It is not enough to assign QA personnel, human factors engineers, and risk managers to the team and expect them to cover all of these areas. The topics are sufficiently important that all team members should be aware of the requirements, as individuals may know of situations that are not apparent to outsiders. In addition, depending on the past history of the company, team building and teamwork training might be very useful. Remember that this training needs to be documented and made a part of the training file for each team member.

The management/administrative team will also have the responsibility to identify and remove structural (organizational) barriers that impede progress in design development. The guideline on Design Control assigns the responsibility for dealing with structural barriers to senior management. Indeed, the presence of many structural barriers in a company is often a sign of a breakdown in senior management. These barriers may arise from the company's culture, environment, or the technology being employed. The usual symptoms are poor communications and a lack of strong interactions among groups whose activities are critical to the development of the device. Some of these barriers can be simple things such as the lack of clear instructions assigning responsibilities for different areas of design development.

Personnel do not need to be restricted to particular subteams. Except for the individual designated by the regulations for the design review group, other individuals may serve in more than one subteam. In the case of small companies this will probably be a requirement, and in larger companies it may be dictated by factors such as specialized training or by an individual's special knowledge of a particular type of device or subject.

The whole project team must remain intact throughout the life cycle of the device. The requirement for modifications throughout the life cycle of the device means that while the team may fluctuate in size and personnel, its basic elements must remain to deal with changes and, possibly, to develop any successor to the original device.

Note that if the manufacturer contracts with a specification developer to develop the initial specifications for the device, the specification developer is also subject to the design control regulations.

Note also that if design changes are made to existing devices, including those that were licensed before the effective date of these CGMP regulations, the changes will be subject to these design control regulations. The document prepared in response to this paragraph should allow for this situation and specify the actions to be taken when design revisions are made to a device that existed before July 1, 1997.

Devices that will be manufactured under an Investigational Device Exemption (IDE) will not be exempt from design controls. The FDA has always required IDE devices to be manufactured under a state of control, and in the preamble to the current CGMP, the FDA announced that it is amending the IDE regulation (21 CFR 812) to state that IDE devices will not be exempt from the design control regulations of 21 CFR 820.30.

Class I devices that appear to be exempt from design control are still subject to 21 CFR 820.181 and must be properly introduced into the production system.

21 CFR 820.30(b) Design and Development Planning. Each manufacturer shall establish and maintain plans that describe or reference the design and development activities and define responsibility for implementation. The plans shall identify and describe the interfaces with different groups or activities that provide, or result in, input to the design and development process. The plans shall be reviewed, updated, and approved as design and development evolves.

16. **Design Development Management.** This management document should be prepared by the management/administrative team and executed in association with the whole project team. The document should contain plans covering the expected design and development activities and an assignment of the activities to departments or to certain specified positions in particular departments. This document should describe the general requirements for planning, including plans for concurrent engineering that will give rise to a design and development plan for a specific device. For large projects, the use of activity network diagrams generated by PERT (Program Evaluation and Review Technique) or CPM (Critical Path Method) or the use of Gantt Charts for scheduling activities, should be considered. It should not apply to devices that are in the conceptual or research stage, where their feasibility has not yet been determined. However, once a decision has been made to proceed with the development of the device, the design and development plan should be produced before further work takes place. It is usually useful to document the sequence of activities that took place during the design development process so that an FDA inspector will know where research ended and development of the device design began. The plans should define and assign the responsibility for their implementation. If necessary, it could be a "how to" document, describing how the design requirements will be addressed and how the design that is released for production will be shown to meet approved requirements. The document should be a broadly applicable document in the sense of defining responsibilities rather than providing exact specifications and production steps. Although the company will probably be focused on design or product development at this point, it should remember that review and verification activities as well as

quality systems and regulatory requirements must be included in this planning. The realities of concurrent engineering and the development of technically complex devices will often call for multiple cycles of design development and evaluation that will continue even after manufacturing has commenced. Therefore the document prepared here must be flexible enough to deal with these situations, and provisions for the periodic review and updating of the document should be made.

The document should clearly address the issues of risk analysis and risk management not only from the point of view of the patient or operator, but also address potential problems in the manufacture of the device. It should specify the tools to be used such as Fault Tree Analysis (FTA) and Failure Mode and Effect Analysis (FMEA). The issue of manufacturing safety should be addressed especially if the design will require the use of hazardous processes or material. The Design Control Guideline is especially helpful in discussing risk management and should be consulted.

The design activity involves not only the development of the device but also the production process, labeling and packaging, and after sales servicing and monitoring. All of these activities need to undergo design development and review and are subject to design control procedures. An example given in the guideline, notes that while a device design may require the product to be sterile, it should also be designed to be sterilizable by the sterilization process that is chosen for manufacturing use. Furthermore the packaging must be designed to maintain the device in a sterile state until it is used and to have some mechanism to warn the user if sterility is violated.

There should be consideration given to interactions among groups and activity areas and a definition of how the interfaces should work. Interfaces, such as those between the Design development team and Marketing, Purchasing, Sales, Manufacturing, Information Systems, Regulatory Affairs, Maintenance, and Field Service, should be defined. The information that will be passed between the groups needs to be defined (who tells what to whom). If any of the interfaces appear to be barriers instead (for instance a document that requires ten reviews and signatures before it can be sent to the next group), the team will need to bring the barrier to the attention of upper management who will be responsible for removing the barrier. The manufacturer's internal structure and the composition of the Design development team will dictate the needs for defined interfaces. Finally, there should be a mechanism for reviewing, updating, and approving the plans as the design and development work evolve.

The design development plan along with the documents generated during the review, updating, and approval of the plans, as they evolve, should become a part of the DHF.

21 CFR 820.30(c) Design Input. *Each manufacturer shall establish and maintain procedures to ensure that the design requirements relating to a device are appropriate and address the intended use of the device, including the needs of the user and patient. The procedures shall include a mechanism for addressing incomplete, ambiguous, or conflicting requirements. The design input requirements shall be documented and shall be reviewed and approved by a designated individual(s). The approval, including the date and signature of the individual(s) approving the requirements, shall be documented.*

21 CFR 820.3(f) Design input *means the physical and performance requirements of a device that are used as a basis for device design.*

17. **Design Input.** This document should assign the responsibility for design input to the design development team who will be responsible for developing and specifying all of the physical and performance requirements that will become design inputs. If the design will be large and complex, it may be necessary to divide the design development team into several subteams that will have the responsibility to design specific aspects of the device. If this happens, each subteam should have a document defining its mission and responsibilities and the group as a whole will need a coordination and administration function to maintain schedules and information flow and resolve conflicting requirements or specifications among the subteams. For a better idea of what should be considered as part of the design input, review the expected components of the design output as noted in 21 CFR 820.3(g). Note that operating, servicing,

and maintenance manuals as well as labeling and packaging in general should be defined in the design output, so design input criteria for these areas should also be present. Labeling, in particular, is critical and a subgroup of the design development team might be assigned to determine the content, composition, and wording of the labels. This subgroup should contain a person familiar with the regulations related to labeling. Other items to be included in the design input should be the requirements for containers used in storing and shipping the devices, the tests or testing that will be required, requirements for maintenance and servicing, and any special equipment that will be required to produce the device.

The design development team should be composed of personnel from all groups responsible for design development such as R & D, Engineering, and so on, and also those groups such as Purchasing and Marketing who have key support functions to perform. The Quality Systems function should be represented along with Regulatory Affairs. These individuals from the supporting groups may be fewer in number than the actual design development personnel, and they need to be experienced in determining the needs of devices. Personnel who lack experience will often allow matters to proceed to a critical juncture and then allow the team to discover a multitude of issues that should have been covered as the development progressed. For this reason, if less experienced workers are assigned to teams, they must be in communication with the more experienced members of their functional groups.

The initial responsibility for providing the original input for the design should lie with the Marketing function. They should be responsible for conducting the market research that will determine customer needs in relation to the device and, for that matter, the need for the device itself. Other sources should also be consulted to determine unstated customer needs and cycles of surveys may be needed to accurately assess customer needs. This is especially true if the nature of the targeted customer population begins to evolve as the company learns more about the capabilities of the device. Technical, medical, regulatory and safety issues must be considered even if they are not explicitly raised in a survey of customer needs. For instance, customers expect a device to be safe to use and to be usable by left- and right-handed operators, but these expectations may not be explicitly expressed or considered by the design team. Also, it makes little sense to design a beautiful, chrome-finished, stainless steel device costing $100 when all the customer wanted was a plastic disposable device costing $3.95. Customer needs should be addressed early in the design development process to minimize the probability that a company will develop a device that the customer does not want. Also, some design inputs may, in turn, create other inputs. A device that must fit on a bedside cart will have certain requirements that will be different from those of a fixed position, washing machine-sized instrument.

Design input consists of the design requirements and the document covering them should have a description of a design input report that will contain a statement of the requirements relative to the needs created by the intended use of the device. The needs created by the intended use of the device should include the needs of the user and patient and would, therefore, include matters such as safety and human factors. The manufacturer must assess and set the levels of safety and efficacy that are in keeping with the intended use of the device. Thus the input should consist of performance characteristics, safety and reliability requirements, physical characteristics, environmental needs, regulatory and other standards, and packaging and labeling requirements. The environmental needs involve defining the environment needed for the device to operate properly or designing the device to meet the customer's environmental needs. Other factors that might be considered when establishing input requirements are energy fields, physical shock, toxicity, biocompatibility, electrostatic discharge, the ability of the device to cope with line voltage fluctuations, and the preservation of programming in the event of an electrical failure or power surge. The regulatory and quality system needs for the device should also be accommodated at this stage.

In the Quality System Manual, reference is made to seven basic design input questions that need to be answered. These questions involve the need and use of the new device and cover the types of questions that a marketing survey should be designed to answer. There is a further discussion of the need for producing an "input checklist" to cope with the large number and complexity of the input requirements. If this checklist is created, it should also be used as a design output checklist. A major problem with this checklist is that it must undergo a wide review and approval process. With a subject as broad and complex as design input, it is easy for requirements to be missed. Once the checklist is created, one can encounter a type of mindless behavior where things not on the list are considered to be unimportant just because they are not on the list. For this reason the checklist must receive a periodic review.

A critical part of the design input will be the configuration management plan. This plan should describe the controlled documents that will constitute and define the design configuration. Typically, these would be specifications, design documents, test documents, and documents required for regulatory records. The document controls, including the system for cross-referencing these documents, should be defined.

Before the input requirements are converted into outputs, a review should be conducted to decide if the inputs generated meet the design needs of the device and are reasonable in the light of manufacturing capabilities and the economics of the product. In addition, the ability of the device to meet competition should be assessed as well as the possibility that the design needs are generating unusual requirements. These would be factors such as new or different regulatory interpretations, or the necessity of developing new testing equipment for the quality control of the device. The regulations require the design input to address incomplete, ambiguous or conflicting requirements. These must be resolved before proceeding. Finally the input statements should be reviewed and approved to be sure that they say what needs to be said in a clear and unambiguous fashion.

As the design development proceeds, there will be a periodic need to update the design input requirements. This will continue even after the device is licensed and on the market. The older versions of the input documents should be placed in the DHF to show the sequence of events that led to more recent designs.

21 CFR 820.30(d) Design Output. *Each manufacturer shall establish and maintain procedures for defining and documenting design output in terms that allow an adequate evaluation of conformance to design input requirements. Design output procedures shall contain or make reference to acceptance criteria and shall ensure that those design outputs that are essential for the proper functioning of the device are identified. Design output shall be documented, reviewed, and approved before release. The approval, including the date and the signature of the individual(s) approving the output, shall be documented.*

21 CFR 820.3(g) Design output *means the results of a design effort at each design phase and at the end of the total design effort. The finished design output is the basis of the device master record. The total finished design output consists of the device, its packaging and labeling, and the device master record.*

18. **Design Output.** This document needs to establish the general responsibilities for the design output. The design output, itself, includes the device and all associated specifications, drawings and accessories such as the packaging and labeling that were produced in response to the design input requirements. The design development team is initially responsible for design output. Having created the input, they should be able to take at least a first cut at providing the appropriate output. This is especially important as the input-output cycle will occur many times over the course of device development and over the life cycle of the device. The design output itself should be documents prepared in response to the requirements that constituted the design input. The input checklist should now become an output checklist. The output must be in terms that will allow for verification or validation (in other words, they should contain specifications and limits for key parameters), and these requirements should have been confirmed through design verification and validation and ensured by design review.

    The design output should be described at the end of each design phase and each design phase should be defined in the design and development plan. An example given by the FDA in their Quality System Manual states that the first design output document will usually be the design requirements document which will contain the preliminary design specifications. This document itself will evolve as the workers develop a better understanding of the design requirements for their device. Based on the Design Control Guideline, the design output should be detailed documentation covering all functional and performance characteristics of the device and the product and process documents needed to produce the device and maintain it throughout its life cycle. They should contain the manufacturing process specifications, the quality assurance/control testing and specifications, and the device packaging and labeling. Design output documents should be things such as laboratory notebooks, scientific and technical reports, verification protocols and data, capability studies and process validations. The design output should consider not just the design itself. It should also consider everything about the device, including safety factors, from the initial decision to develop the design, through manufacturing and distribution, to the end-of-life of the device (for instance, what do you do about a gamma ray source when the irradiation machine becomes obsolete). In addition, the document needs to specify the titles and designations of documents describing or controlling the device packaging; labeling; material, component, and device specifications; production instructions; quality assurance and control procedures; and release criteria for raw material, intermediates, and final products.

When the device might be adversely affected by the process raw materials, equipment, or the process itself, the sources of these potential adverse effects should be identified. Warnings about these adverse effects should be included in the appropriate design output documents, and included in the training of the appropriate employees.

The design output control document should contain a description of review procedures to make sure that the design output documents will meet the requirements of the design input for the stage being studied. Design outputs needed for the proper functioning of the device must be identified, along with the input that led to them. Acceptance criteria and the procedures for measuring them must be specified in the appropriate documents. The acceptance criteria should be shown to satisfy the needs of specific parts of the design input. One of the problems encountered here arises from the fact that during the early stages of development, the development team may not have a clear idea of what constitutes a good specification. As a result there is a tendency to set specifications that say things like, "greater than X units." The problem is that a part that has 2X units may be acceptable, but a part that has 100X units will be completely unacceptable due to physical limitations alone. When setting limit specifications, it is usually better to set an interval rather than a specific number. Specific numbers will work with "less than" specifications but "at least" and "more than" specifications should have an upper limit even if it is so high as to seem ridiculous.

Note that, while the design input may stay the same, the output may change as different methods or materials are used to meet the input requirements. Thus the design output may evolve as production develops. This creates a need for mechanisms to control, review, and approve new or modified outputs. The manufacturer may begin the production process before all design activities are completed, but all design specifications that are released to the production group must be approved and verified or validated through the design output process before they can be implemented. All of these documents, as well as those mentioned above, must be included in the DHF.

The information and specifications listed in 21 CFR 820.181 as components of the Device Master Record (DMR) are the types of material that are expected to be seen in the design output. In fact the DMR should be regarded as the primary design output. The DMR should include all of the design documentation that is required for production of the device by the manufacturing unit.

19. **Design Output Control.** The design output must be written, reviewed, and approved before release from the design team. The approval must be documented and include the names and dated signatures of the employees responsible for approving the output.

   The design output must be controlled, and before any output is generated a control plan needs to be instituted. The plan should be built around information and documentation flow diagrams that will show where the information and documentation is generated, where it is transmitted, how it is used, and where it is stored. In general, the documentation, including the most recent copies of the device configuration, should be stored where they are used, but backup copies should be maintained in the document control unit. Changes to documents are documented, reviewed, and approved by the same function that approved the original documents. In addition to the copies that are stored at the point of use, the documents should be controlled by a central documentation group that will be responsible for document change control for the DMR, the DHR, and the DHF. This document should establish the control system.

20. **Device Configuration.** This is established by the design output. The configuration management plan that was developed under the design input requirement should be used to control the output. During the design process, design criteria are established as the designers complete engineering diagrams, flow charts, source code, and so on. Before others use these documents they should be formally accepted and recognized as being a part of the device configuration, and then released. As with all other documentation, control is needed to ensure that all parts of the design team are working from the same revision of a particular document. For the purposes of the DHF, this document establishing the device configuration should also specify the location and responsibility for maintaining any physical models leading to the final device and its components. Documents that are recognized as a part of the device configuration should cross-reference each other. This is because different parts of the configuration will interact with each other and a change to one document may easily affect the contents of another. The location and responsibility for maintaining drawings of the final device and all intermediate designs of the device or its components, and for maintaining examples of the packaging and labeling, and any intermediate designs used during the development of the device should be specified.

Device specifications are a part of the device configuration and arise from design inputs. It is important to have forward and backward traceability to ensure that the specifications and the design inputs are clearly connected. Quality Function Deployment (QFD) is a method for ensuring the coupling of specifications with requirements, and it or a similar procedure should be considered for employment in this situation.

21 CFR 820.30(e) Design Review.　 *Each manufacturer shall establish and maintain procedures to ensure that formal documented reviews of the design results are planned and conducted at appropriate stages of the device's design development. The procedures shall ensure that participants at each design review include representatives of all functions concerned with the design stage being reviewed and an individual(s) who does not have direct responsibility for the design stage being reviewed, as well as any specialists needed. The results of a design review, including identification of the design, the date, and the individual(s)performing the review, shall be documented in the design history file (the DHF).*

　21 CFR 820.3(h) Design review *means a documented, comprehensive, systematic examination of a design to evaluate the adequacy of the design requirements, to evaluate the capability of the design to meet these requirements, and to identify problems.*

21. **Design Review Team.** This should be established as a part of the Product Development or Project Team. An individual or group should be identified and given the responsibility for reviewing all documents and actions that result from design input requirements. This team will have the responsibility for conducting the verification and validation activities required by 21 CFR 820.30(f) and (g), for reviewing the correctness of the translation of design outputs into production specifications and directions as required by 21 CFR 820.30(h), and for participating in the review and approval of design changes as required in 21 CFR 820.30(i). This team should also have the ultimate responsibility for configuration management as described in the Design Control Guideline. The review should cover performance, safety, compatibility with other devices, overall system requirements, human factors, and environmental compatibility.

　　This team should be composed of representatives from the same groups that were represented on the design development team with additional personnel from the quality systems and regulatory functions. In particular, personnel from manufacturing, production and quality assurance will be needed to provide continuity and monitoring as the design proceeds from concept to manufactured product. These people could be the same people who were on the other teams, but the regulations specifically state that management must assign at least one person who does not have direct responsibility for design stage under review to participate in the design review. It is suggested that this individual should be the head of the design review team, and, if possible, members of the design review team should not also be on the design development team. Also, it would seem wise to ensure that no member of the design review team be subordinate to any member of the design development team.

22. **Design Review Team Activities.** The next document should assign and describe the activities of the design review team. This will be a formal design review program that will be delegated to the Design Review Team. The Design Control Guidelines refer to a program of formal meetings that occur throughout the design process. It describes the intent of the design review process as being intended to (1) provide a systematic assessment of the device and associated designs, including accessories, components, software, labeling, packaging, production, installation and service, production and support; (2) provide feedback to designers on existing or emerging problems; (3) assess project progress; and (4) provide confirmation that the project is ready to move on to the next stage of development. The names and departmental positions and affiliations of the individuals participating in the reviews should be recorded. Also, for the benefit of later workers, the minutes or a summary of the group discussions should be included in the report from each design review meeting. There should also be a requirement that all members of the reviewing group who approve of the results of the design review sign and date the report. This is preferable to a single signature by the leader of the group, as it will help approving members to assume responsibility for the design. There should also be a requirement for a review of the adequacy of design input requirements as the design evolves.

These documents as well as the document that establishes the requirements for this part shall be included in the DHF.

23. **Design Review Control.** The next document needed here is one that will control the design reviews themselves. Taking into account the requirements of document 22, it should contain directions for conducting a design review, and a statement on when the reviews should be performed. These formal reviews must be performed at specified stages and the directions should not contain generalities such as "as needed" or "at appropriate stages." These should be requirements for periodic design reviews during device development and after a product is licensed and in full production, especially if significant complaints or servicing problems arise. The review needs to be comprehensive for the design phase that is being studied and should show that the design satisfies design input requirements but does not need to be comprehensive for the complete design process. It should review the design verification and validation activities to determine if the design will perform properly, is compatible with its accessories, and meets requirements for reliability and other factors considered as part of the design input. There should also be a requirement to list the names, positions, and functional affiliations of all participants in the design review. These individuals should be technically qualified to perform the review. Another provision should be included to allow the team to be modified for particular types of meetings by allowing additional, invited, representation from affected departments.

The regulations require these reviews to be documented and for the documents to become a part of the DHF. The point to remember here is that the design will need to evolve as new materials, subassemblies, and techniques become available. Also, customer or user needs may change and create a need for new design inputs. Consequently, the design review report should identify any problems noted during the review. The design review does not need to contain proposed solutions to the problems, but should contain a requirement that solutions be found.

21 CFR 820.30(f) Design Verification. *Each manufacturer shall establish and maintain procedures for verifying the device design. De-*

sign verification shall confirm that the design output meets the design input requirements. The results of the design verification, including identification of the design, method(s), the date, and the individual(s) performing the verification shall be documented in the DHF.

21 CFR 820.3(aa) Verification *means confirmation by examination and provision of objective evidence that specified requirements have been fulfilled.*

Design Control Guideline: *Design verification is confirmation that design output meets design input requirements. . . . Globally, design verification is the process by which conformance to design specifications is confirmed and the question "did we design the device right" is answered. Locally, verification is the process by which the output of a design activity is evaluated to determine conformity with the input requirement for that activity.*

21 CFR 820.30(f), Design Verification and Validation, actually creates a need for several documents, all of which must be placed in the DHF. The results of these verification activities, including an identification of the design and device reviewed, methods used, date, and the name(s) of the individual(s) who performed the verification should be entered into a report and the report should become a part of the DHF.

24. **Design Verification Activities.** The first is a design verification review document defining the specific responsibilities of the design review team for verifying that the specific design output meets the requirements of the design input. The need for this document arises because the design output can occur in many forms, and it may not be possible for one group to be aware of design output activities in another group. Consequently, a design verification activity document should be created to describe a review that is conducted to confirm that design output documents were prepared to address all of the design inputs, and that the documents were executed with required actions taken and reports prepared. This document should be coordinated with the documents prepared for 21 CFR 820.30(d).

    The qualification of components, including software validation, should be a part of the verification activity, and separate documents may be needed to direct activities that will show that components will meet the design requirements. Actual qualification testing, as opposed to accepting catalogue specifications, may need to be performed.

If prototypes are used in clinical trials, they should be subjected to design verification for safety to the maximum extent possible. However, prototypes are not necessarily identical to the device that will be produced in actual manufacturing runs. Final design verification, which may include clinical trials, therefore must include testing of actual production-derived devices under actual or simulated conditions of use and in the actual or simulated environment. Note that devices that fall under "substantial equivalency" rules may not have to go through clinical trials. However, the complexity of devices and the regulatory situation make it imperative that the manufacturer discuss this with CDRH and not assume that the device is exempt.

The design verification process is controlled by (1) ensuring that device specifications are verifiable and traceable to requirements of design inputs, (2) planning and systematically verifying design outputs as being traceable to the design specifications, and (3) using the design review process to determine if the verification activities themselves are appropriate, consistent, complete, and traceable. The Design Control Guideline goes on to state that verification activities are planned and that they include testing, inspection, analysis, review, etc. Among the things that need to be reviewed are the results of Failure Mode Effect Analysis (FMEA), Fault Tree Analysis (FTA), and other risk analyses. These analyses should consider an instrument in normal and fault conditions, that is, if a fault is present, can it lead to another fault? These analyses can also be redone to verify the removal of hazards or potentially hazardous situations, especially when the extremes of operating conditions are considered. When manufacturing begins, procedures for testing and accepting incoming, in-process, and final products should be validated and in place.

It is possible that *in vitro* testing alone will not be sufficient to verify the design of a device. Animal or clinical testing may be required. The Design Control Guidelines state that animal testing must precede clinical testing, and animal testing is done only after (a) it can be shown that *in vitro* testing alone is insufficient to verify certain aspects of the design, and (b) *in vitro* testing has, as much as possible, shown that the product is safe and satisfactory.

In addition to these reviews, the labeling of the instrument needs to be verified from the user's perspective. The device should be run so that all labeling, screen displays, and other outputs may be observed and verified. The labeling and screen displays should match what is expected on the basis of the operator's manual and the requirements of the design output. This review should also apply to any printouts that are generated by the device. The information in the printouts, especially patient identification, should be reviewed to ensure that a person who is technically qualified, but new to the particular patient's situation will be able to understand the printout. The FDA has stated that the labeling is often directed to the manufacturer's needs and that the user's needs may be forgotten. One might expect the FDA to be concerned about this situation when they review the verification.

If there are conflicts or problems, the group or individual designated as the design review team should have the authority to initiate action to correct the situation. Since design output monitoring and updating are activities that should be maintained throughout the manufacturing life of the product, the group or individual named here may change or evolve as the product moves through development and into production, but the team must remain in existence.

The procedures developed for the design verification, validation, or review are potential procedures for QC and QA activities. They should be reviewed with this in mind, and appropriate validation activities should be scheduled to allow the procedures to be used for QA/QC examination of the device.

21 CFR 820.30(g) Design Validation. *Each manufacturer shall establish and maintain procedures for validating the device design. Design validation shall be performed under defined operating conditions on initial production units, lots, or batches, or their equivalents. Design validation shall ensure that devices conform to defined user needs and intended uses and shall include testing of* *production units under actual or simulated use conditions. Design validation shall include software validation and risk analysis, where appropriate. The results of the design validation, including identification of the design, method(s), the date, and the individual(s) performing the validation, shall be documented in the DHF.*

21 CFR 820.3(z) Validation *means confirmation by examination and provision of objective evidence that the particular requirements for a specific intended use can be consistently fulfilled.*

21 CFR 820.3(z)(2) Design Validation *means establishing by objective evidence that device specifications conform with user needs and intended use(s).*

Design Control Guideline: *The intent of design validation is to go beyond the purely technical issues of verifying that the design output meets the design input, and is intended to ensure that the device meets user requirements. Conceptually, device validation is performed with respect to the design input requirements and answers the question, "Did we design the right device?"*

25. **Design Validation Protocol.** This document needs to establish a procedure of planning for the validation with a statement of procedures to be used and criteria to be met. The planning procedure itself needs to be reviewed to assure that the validation study will be appropriate and complete. The validation may involve testing under both actual and simulated use conditions and the planning for the validation will need to evolve as the design evolves. The FDA has stated, in the preamble to the Quality System regulations, that design verification is not a substitute for design validation. As the defined user needs and intended uses should have been a part of the design input requirements, the validation must show that the finished device, as manufactured, does satisfy those device input requirements and that there has been proper overall design control and proper design transfer. (Note that this is a review of the actual finished device and not just a review of documents.) This is a validation on the early units, lots or batches of a new design, possibly at the pilot production level. It is not a release protocol. The validation should be under simulated use conditions to satisfy the requirement that the device will be suitable for its

intended use. To this end, a clinical evaluation of the device may become an important component of the design validation.

The design verification is performed against specifications that the manufacturer will have developed during the design development process. As such, some of these specifications will be present mainly to meet the needs of the manufacturer. In contrast the design validation is performed to validate the device's ability to satisfy user needs and intended uses. It is important to remember that there may be more than one intended user. With medical devices it is often important to consider the needs of clinicians in addition to the patient. In fact the clinicians may be the real users with the patient being simply the recipient of the actions of the device.

It is possible that it may be necessary to use an "equivalent" or surrogate device in the validation study. While this may be allowed, the FDA will want to see detailed documentation on how the surrogate was produced. The documentation should also discuss how the surrogate is similar to and also different from a device that would be manufactured during initial production runs on the manufacturer's premises. An analysis of the differences will become very important in the situation where an "equivalent" device is used under simulated conditions. As might be expected, the question of how "equivalent" the surrogate is will have a bearing on the validity of this type of validation.

In the Design Control Guideline it was suggested that if possible, the design validation should be performed by an independent team familiar with the details of the project but not directly involved in the design process. Initially, it appeared that this team could be the Design Review Team, but, in many ways, members of this team will be actively involved with the design process, if they are doing their jobs. On the other hand, with a new product and appropriate security considerations, it may be difficult to find additional qualified individuals who are familiar with project details but not actively involved with the design process. For this reason, a good compromise may be to use the Design Review Team, but to augment it with selected individuals from the user community. These individuals should be able to provide the independent perspective required for a good validation study.

26. **Software Evaluation.** A protocol should be prepared for any software validation that needs to be done. This will need to be done for any software that is required for the proper functioning of the device. If the software is a well-known or a frequently reviewed package, it may be sufficient to name the software, to name its publisher, and to demonstrate that it is capable of performing the functions needed by the device. For programming that was developed specifically for the device, it may be necessary to write out the code and have an independent reviewer verify that the programming will perform its intended function. Finally, the device's programming should be validated under conditions of use by observing or reviewing the device's performance to show that functions that are programming-dependent do perform as expected even with extreme or aberrant inputs to the programming. Software validation should include questions related to hardware failures. It is important to know how the software will cope with disconnected lines, a jammed motor, static charges, and so on.

Just because the programming was correct, it does not mean that the programming will be installed correctly. There are FDA and ISO guidance documents available that will help in software validation and software risk analysis. Risk analysis must be performed for the software and it may be necessary to obtain help from external sources to perform appropriate FMEA and FTA studies. The risk analysis on the software should be coordinated with the activities in the next document (27).

If there are one or more software packages that are critical to the design or manufacturing of the device (e.g., Computer Assisted Design or Computer Assisted Manufacturing (CAD/CAM) program packages), the software should be validated by means of a validation protocol. If the program is widely distributed or has been in use over a long time so that defects or operating problems are well known, it will be sufficient to show that the software is capable of functioning properly for its intended use. If the program is locally written or custom made for the production of the device, it may be necessary to conduct a full, detailed validation. An independent reviewer such as a software consulting group may be the best for this situation. Even if you have purchased a copy of a well-known software package, this does not guarantee that your copy (a) does not contain a random error in the form of an electronic "bug," (b) was properly installed into your computer, or (c) that you or your staff know how to use it properly. The validation protocol should consider these possibilities and address each one in turn. The computer itself may create a need for periodic revalidations. If the configuration and interaction between the computer and program are such that limitations due to memory or communications port allocations are becoming critical, functional problems may arise if additional programs are loaded into the computer or if the allocation of resources among programs is changed. For these reasons, software packages should undergo at least a simple validation study on a periodic basis and when major changes are made to the software or hardware configuration of the computer. Refer to 21 CFR 820.70(i) for other software-related regulations and procedures that overlap with this regulation. This document (26) and document 54 will need to be coordinated.

27. **Risk Analysis.** The final document needed to satisfy the requirements of 21 CFR 820.30(g) will be a protocol to evaluate the device for potential sources of harm to the patient or operator. At the validation stage these studies should be conducted on the actual device or a prototype unit that is very close to the actual device that will be manufactured. The protocol should analyze the available information not only to note the potential sources of harm, but also to estimate the probable rate of occurrence and the degree of severity of the harmful event. The manufacturer will be expected to identify potential hazards associated with the device in normal and fault conditions. Any hazard that is deemed unacceptable should be reduced to acceptable levels. A major part of this assessment will be to identify the various possible fault conditions and their causes. FMEA and FTA should be a part of this risk analysis. If

there are plans for external evaluations of the device's safety, such as Underwriters Laboratories or CSA certifications, these studies and their protocols should become a part of this activity. A Certified Reliability Engineer will prove useful here.

21 CFR 820.30(h) Design Transfer. *Each manufacturer shall establish and maintain procedures to ensure that the device design is correctly translated into production specifications.*

Design Control Guideline: *The transfer of a device design to production typically involved review and approval of specifications, procedures, and critical product and process characteristics established in the FMEAs, FTAs, and hazard analyses. Where applicable, it includes confirmation of the adequacy of specifications, methods, and procedures through process validation, including the reliability and durability testing of finished product under actual or simulated use conditions.*

28. **Design Transfer.** Basically, the design transfer document should describe a series of reviews that will compare production specifications and processing activities to design requirements as given in the design output to verify that the production documents as written do satisfy the needs of the design.

    Where a process is involved, these would be process validation or product validation studies that show that the device and its manufacturing process meets the design requirements. These studies should confirm the device specifications and production methods and procedures. The FDA no longer has an absolute requirement for studies on three consecutive production runs, but it continues to feel that three production runs during process validations is the accepted standard. Each production specification will need its own confirmation, and a responsible individual will need to review and approve the production specifications to ensure that all of the pertinent design requirements are being met by the production specifications. In turn, these studies could result in an actual fabrication of subassemblies under simulated or actual manufacturing conditions. The procedures used would be reviewed and examined to ensure that what is manufactured is what was intended. Eventually, these subunits would be assembled into actual devices that would be used in the validation studies of 21 CFR 820.30(g). These reviews could be viewed as approval procedures for production specifications, or process procedures and documented as such. Also, these activities would allow an evaluation of the actual utility of purchased parts and material and allow an evaluation of the adequacy of the specifications used for their purchase.

The ultimate goal of these activities is to ensure the correct translation of design output requirements into manufacturing directions and specifications. The directions should be designed to produce a product that meets the related specifications. The specifications, in turn, should be shown to meet customer needs. These translations need to occur within the context of the manufacturer's document change control system.

21 CFR 820.30(i) Design Changes. Each manufacturer shall establish and maintain procedures for the identification, documentation, validation, or where appropriate, verification, review, and approval of design changes before their implementation.

Design Control Guideline: *Configuration management refers to the documentation to be controlled, the procedures for controlling it, and the responsibilities of those managing the documentation, i.e., the configuration control board. It includes a system of traceability including traceability of components, service manuals, procedures, etc. that could be affected by a change. The controlled documents are configuration items and collectively form the device configuration.*

Typically, the device configuration includes specifications, design documents, test documents, and all other deliverables, including those documents required for regulatory records.

29. **Design Change Control.** If the design of a device is regarded as an evolving construct that will change even after licensed production is begun, the preceding requirements for design review, verification, and validation will lead to the proper actions being taken when changes occur, and design changes can be accommodated within the existing framework that requires documented and approved changes.

    The document covering design change control should require a statement on the nature of the configuration and documents to be controlled, and situations when change control is required. The change control process should evaluate the change to see if other documents or procedures will be affected by the change. Part of this document should define significant and nonsignificant design changes with instructions on the actions to be taken and the need for a review to determine which changes are significant and which are not. The actual document covering a particular change should contain a statement on the reason for the change, and the effects that the change is expected to have on the process or finished product. The change itself must be evaluated to see if it will require the submission of a 510(k) according to 21 CFR 807.81(a)(3) or if a PMA supplement needs to be made following 21 CFR 814.39. Even if neither of these actions is required, a record of the evaluation and its results should be made.

The remaining requirements will be covered by the document change control system that the manufacturer should have established already. Basically, this document needs to make a statement on how design changes are to be accommodated. A decision on how the design change is to be checked also is required. As usual, if the change cannot be verified by inspection or testing, it will need to be validated. It is important to know if the basic design configuration will be maintained or if the change will result in a new configuration.

The documents generated by the design control activities of this part must be considered to be controlled documents and subject to the requirements of 21 CFR 820.40. This document must specify the approval process that design changes must undergo before they, and their documentation, are accepted and incorporated into the system.

30. **Configuration Management.** A very important control document must be prepared here. The Design Review Team and the Documentation group must be assigned the responsibility for configuration management. Depending on a firm's existing structure, the configuration control group could be the Design Review Team or an existing Change Control Board or a completely new creation such as a configuration management team. The activities of the configuration management team

must be defined in this document. A large part of the responsibility will fall on the documentation system. An electronic system featuring many keywords and document indices will prove its worth the first time a major change must be made. As the design matures and production procedures become fixed, the consequences of a change will become more severe and the importance of configuration management will increase.

A major problem here is that design changes will not just cause document changes. These changes can result in the necessity for additional work on the device itself with associated changes in other documents that constitute the configuration of the device. As an example, consider a design change that leads to a change in a raw material specification, a processing procedural document, and a final product specification. In turn this could lead to a need for a new raw material acceptance test procedure, a new in-process inspection procedure, and a new final product acceptance test. Since this changes the configuration, new data will be needed for regulatory submissions, and a major change could invalidate previous preclinical or clinical studies. Thus the configuration management team will need to be familiar with the whole manufacturing process as well as the device design itself.

※ Subpart D—Document Controls ※

21 CFR 820.40 Document Controls

Each manufacturer shall establish and maintain procedures to control all documents that are required by this part. The procedures shall provide for the following:

21 CFR 820.40(a) Document Approval and Distribution.

Each manufacturer shall designate an individual(s) to review for adequacy and approve prior to issuance all documents established to meet the requirements of this part. The approval, including the date and signature of the individual(s) approving the document, shall be documented. Documents established to meet the requirements of this part shall be available at all locations for which they are designated, used, or otherwise necessary, and all obsolete documents shall be promptly removed from all points of use or otherwise prevented from unintended use.

31. **Document Control Unit.** First of all, if the manufacturer does not have one already, a documentation unit needs to be established. This unit will be responsible for the whole documentation system as described in the Introduction in Part I. Establishing a unit responsible for the documentation system must be coordinated with the formation of the records group needed for 21 CFR 820.180. In fact, the considerations required for meeting the requirements of 21 CFR 820.180 should be incorporated into this document, covering 21 CFR 820.40(a) in such a way that the requirements of 21 CFR 820.40 and 21 CFR 820.180 can be met with one group of employees. In addition to the usual administrative details of the reporting relationships, the unit should be assigned the responsibility of maintaining and storing all documents and back-up copies, establishing a standard format for each type of document, maintaining a document classification system, routing all documents and document changes for approval, and storing all changes and versions of documents. The unit should also be given review and approval authority to verify that all documents are in the proper format, have been properly reviewed and approved, and meet basic standards for language and document structure. The unit should also have the responsibility for distributing documents to all appropriate locations, for controlling the distribution of the documents to specified locations, and for removing and destroying all obsolete documents, except for copies maintained for historical reasons. This unit should prepare and maintain indices for the DHR, DHF, and DMR.

  The classification of documents is very important. It may not seem important to a small company, but as the company grows, document classification will be needed to control the huge amount of paper circulating throughout the company. All documents do not need to be present in all company locations. The documents present in a given location should be those needed by the department or individuals to accomplish their work. Documents irrelevant for a department's or individual's functions should not be circulated through these locations. At the very least, the classification of documents will reduce the amount of paper circulating and will help to maintain security even in network based systems.

A documentation system based on a computer network is useful, because document review, approval, and updating can occur quickly. However, this can turn into a nightmare if the wrong documentation system is chosen by the manufacturer. Selection of the software should be done very carefully, as more than just the cost of the software is at stake. The control document should specify the use of passwords and authorization levels to provide security for the documents. These controls should extend not only to document levels but also to document classes. With computer-based systems, it is very important to control the printing of documents or the proliferation of prints and photocopies will result in the bypassing of the system, rendering document control ineffective. It is very important to control document changes and limit access to the core of original documents. Allowing employees to work for long periods with redlined or other locally modified documents is sloppy management and will eventually lead to a breakdown of the document control system.

For archival purposes, a printed copy of all documents along with the changes and all justifications and authorizations for the changes will need to be held in a file specific to each document. This file should show the evolution of the document through all issues since the original was prepared. The reasons for each document change should also be noted, along with the approvals given. Signatures, including electronic "signatures," of approvers should be recorded. Copies of these documents will need to be stored in a safe place. If, through the use of scanners, all of this can be computerized, a secure duplicate copy of all of the electronic material still must be held in a safe location, usually at a remote site. These copies of documents and the storage system should play a role in the company's disaster recovery plan.

32. **Document Distribution.** The documentation unit, having been given the authority to control the distribution and location

of the documents, needs a document to specify how this is to happen and what control mechanisms will be used. A part of this document should establish procedures for establishing a "document location." This might be a simple procedure by which a person or department could ask to receive all documents of a certain class or from several classes. This person or department would then be specified as a document location for documents in those classes. Security and related considerations say that at least one supervisory individual should review and approve any request for document access.

New document approval can be handled as a part of the document change control system. The new document is regarded as a change from nothing and handled the same way as a changed document. Perhaps a notation that the document is new could be made.

The distribution and retrieval of documents must be carefully done, as it is easy to overlook a document held by a sick worker or at a remote location. Electronic systems are preferred, because the document can be deleted and replaced on a specified day without the necessity of physical delivery and retrieval. Departments should use secondary systems to ensure that current documents are used at all times. For instance in the QC laboratory, the analyst could be required to record the effective date of a document or its version number on the result reporting form. A similar procedure could be employed in manufacturing areas.

The unit that performs internal quality auditing (see 21 CFR 820.22) should be responsible for verifying the presence of current documents and the removal of obsolete documents from departments, during an audit of the document control unit. This whole issue will be a major problem for the document control unit. If the company uses a system of distributing printed copies of documents, it is probably best to have a document clerk actually walk around and issue the new document while retrieving the old from the locations or individuals who have been designated as document locations. It is almost impossible to prevent employees from using photocopies of the primary document and then working from a marked-up copy. It is only by a strong educational effort that a company can maintain the integrity of its documentation system. Auditors looking for non-conformances often pick the documentation system as a target because it is usually easy to find an employee working from an obsolete document.

21 CFR 820.40(b) Document Changes. *Changes to documents shall be reviewed and approved by an individual(s) in the same function or organization that performed the original review and approval, unless specifically designated otherwise. Approved changes shall be communicated to the appropriate personnel in a timely manner. Each manufacturer shall maintain records of changes to documents. Change records shall include a description of the change, identification of the affected documents, the signature of the approving individual(s), the approval date, and when the change becomes effective.*

33. **Document Change Control.** Depending upon the company, document change control may be an upper level function that involves managers and supervisors of major functional areas. As mentioned above, the approval and distribution of a new document should follow the same mechanism as that used for changing existing documents. If the document change results from a production or process change, as in 21 CFR 820.70(b), there will be a need for validation or verification of the results of the change before the document can be changed. In many larger companies, document change control follows a two-step process.

In the first step, the document should be routed for approval by supervisors or managers of specific functional or cross-functional areas that will be affected by the change. The procedure document should specify that the document under review must be submitted to managers or supervisors of all affected areas. While a document's originator may specify the reviewers for a new or changed document, the procedure should provide the originator with guidelines on how the reviewers are to be chosen. With a revision of an existing document, the document's file should be consulted to see which groups reviewed the last version of the document. The document should then be reviewed by supervisors or managers from these groups; except, if a group will no longer be affected by the document, the group could be eliminated from the review, if that fact and the reason for it are recorded. If a new group will be affected by the document, that group should be added to the review. Also, it is very important for the originator of a change to identify all other documents that will be affected by the change. If the company does not have a cross-indexing system, major problems can arise when a document is changed, while workers using related documents are not aware of the fact. In one company, a large number of burned-out devices were returned from the field because a specification change for a power supply had not been communicated to workers installing a printed circuit board. The new power supply allowed power surges that could not be tolerated by the printed circuit board. When the specifications for the printed circuit board were changed to compensate for those of the power supply, the problem was corrected, but not before the manufacturer received a large number of returns and created a number of irate customers.

Depending on circumstances, a document could be passed from manager to manager sequentially for review, or multiple copies could be sent out simultaneously for review by all groups. Considerations include the time required for the review and the amount of paper that will be consumed by the simultaneous distribution of a document. This initial review should have strict time limits set for its completion. A maximum of one week should be allotted for each group to perform its review, regardless of whether the document is approved or rejected. For a company with a networked documentation system, a week should be ample time for distribution, review, and retrieval of the document. Supervisors who are traveling, ill, or on vacation should have backup personnel assuming their functions. It is foolish to allow a situation to develop where an individual, through inaction, blocks all progress on a document and its associated changes. If the document is rejected, the reason for the rejection must be stated with a description of what changes would make the document acceptable. The document should be tracked by the document control unit, who should periodically issue status reports on the status of various documents that are in the review process. These status reports should note documents that are overdue and note which groups are holding the documents. The purpose of these reports is to identify the tardy groups and localize the responsibility for the delayed implementation of the documents.

After the review by the affected functional or operational groups, the document should then receive a second review by supervisory personnel who are responsible for broad functions in the company; typically these would include manufacturing, QA/QC, regulatory, marketing, engineering, and scheduling. If desired, a second procedural document could be written here to describe the activities of this second group. All documents, whether approved or rejected, should receive this second review. The purpose of this second review is actually to provide upper management with a chance to monitor and control the changes occurring in a manufacturing site. At this stage, documents may still be rejected. Rejected documents should be returned to the originator with reasons for the rejection and recommendations for making the document acceptable or with a statement that the document or change is unacceptable under all circumstances with reasons given for this conclusion. This second group should not be able to override a rejection by the primary group, but should be able to suggest ways that the rejection could be changed into an acceptance. In the case of serious disagreements over a change, the members of this second reviewing group should be in a position to resolve disputes among the managers or supervisors of the functional groups.

This second group is often known as a Change Control Board (CCB) as the document changes are actually reflecting changes in the company's activities and policies. Therefore the CCB is usually composed of senior managers and has responsibilities that extend to all changes that may affect manufacturing procedures and policies.

Many companies use a standardized cover sheet for document review and describe it in the procedural document for document change control. The cover sheet is usually about two pages long and should include the document name; document control number; document change control tracking number; names and numbers of other affected documents, if any; names of primary reviewing groups, with spaces for dates and signatures of individuals assigned to the review, also with a box or blank for an approval or rejection; a space for a brief summary of the change or a reference to attachments; a space for entering objections that lead to the rejection or in the case of a contingent approval, the requirements for approval to be granted; and, finally, the action taken by the second reviewing group and the signatures or those responsible for the final approval or rejection.

The issue of the effective date for the document or the change could be settled by simply setting a number of days following the date of approval by the second reviewing group. This lead time should be based on the time needed for processing and distributing the document. It should be set by the document control unit. Except for emergency changes (redlining), a change at the workplace should not become effective until the new documents are distributed and are available. Remember that the FDA requires these changes to be communicated to affected personnel "in a timely manner."

The document control unit should keep copies of obsolete documents with copies of the change control documents. The idea is to have a historical record to show what changes have occurred and for what reason.

34. **Temporary Changes.** While 21 CFR 820.40 and its associated documents address document changes, there are several other types of documents closely related to these document change control documents. These are temporary change notices, deviation notices, concessions, redlined documents and so on. These documents are usually generated in response to short-term changes in the ability of the manufacturer to meet certain documented requirements. Sometimes these deviations may be innocuous such as in a case where a procedure is used before its effective date or a lot number is used out of its normal sequence. Others can create major problems. Consider the case where a deviation notice is issued and accepted for a component that has not been tested or inspected. What happens when, after the component has been used to manufacture the device, it is then found that it cannot pass the component's acceptance testing? Another major problem that can arise is where one or more departments work with documents that contain different

procedures or specifications from those used by the rest of the company. The use of redlined documents often leads to these situations because employees are often slow to convert the "redlines" into document changes.

Temporary changes usually involve short-term changes from documented procedures and are essentially temporary changes in the documents themselves. This means that the original documents themselves should be approved and present in the system. Documents that evolve, such as those generated during the design and process development stages should be controlled to a limited extent and placed in the Design History File (DHF) as a record of the stages in the development of the device. They will also show the level of control that existed during the device development process. The temporary change or deviation must be reviewed and approved (usually on an emergency basis) by personnel who are familiar with the area affected by the change. The reason for requiring approval is that there should be some supervisory level agreement that the change will not result in a violation of the license requirements, produce an unsafe product, or create a safety hazard for manufacturing employees. These changes are usually noted on fairly short forms and the approvals may occur without extensive review because of the temporary and emergency nature of the change. If the temporary change affects production or processing as noted in 21 CFR 820.70(b), it may be necessary to introduce and document special verification activities to show that the temporary change did not have an adverse impact on the product that was being made. As the change was temporary, validation of the changed process or production method will not be practical. Repeated or prolonged use of deviation notices may be viewed by auditors or inspectors as an attempt to avoid validations, and the practice should be discouraged.

These temporary changes should have their own format and should be processed in a manner analogous to regular document changes, with allowances being made for the need for haste. The information in these notices should be the same as that required by this part of the regulations for document changes. They should be initiated and routed by the unit that must deal with the change so that the approval or disapproval will be known directly. The deviation notice or a copy should be routed to the document control group, who will place a copy of the notice in all affected product files. Since the need for the deviation notice existed, it should be noted, even if the change was ultimately disapproved. These notices should be monitored so that a unit or process that generates an unusual number or pattern of temporary changes will be noticed by management and the cause of the changes investigated.

❧ Subpart E—Purchasing Controls ❧

21 CFR 820.50 Purchasing Controls

Each manufacturer shall establish and maintain procedures to ensure that all purchased or otherwise received product and services conform to specified requirements.

21 CFR 820.50(a) Evaluation of Suppliers, Contractors, and Consultants. *Each manufacturer shall establish and maintain the requirements, including quality requirements, that must be met by suppliers, contractors, and consultants. Each manufacturer shall:*

(1) *Evaluate and select potential suppliers, contractors, and consultants on the basis of their ability to meet specified requirements, including quality requirements. The evaluation shall be documented.*
(2) *Define the type and extent of control to be exercised over the product, services, suppliers, contractors, and consultants, based on the evaluation results.*
(3) *Establish and maintain records of acceptable suppliers, contractors, and consultants.*

35. **Vendor Approval.** A procedural document is required here to set forth a policy stating that all suppliers, contractors, and consultants that provide material, services, or information critical to the design, manufacturing, or distribution of the device should be evaluated for their ability to meet the manufacturer's needs. This evaluation must occur regardless of the relationship between the supplier and the manufacturer. Other divisions or subdivisions of the manufacturer's company must be

evaluated as if they were independent companies. Preferably, this activity will occur before the vendor's product is purchased or contracts are signed. A distinction between critical and noncritical products and services should be made. The policy should state the need for these evaluations and require the company's purchasing function to avoid major purchases of critical goods or services from firms that are not on the company's list of approved vendors. This document should establish a list of critical supplies and services and of approved vendors. The responsibility for maintaining the list and entering or removing items or organizations from the list should be stated, including a requirement for a periodic review of the vendor's ability to meet the manufacturer's requirements.

The list should show products and services, and the vendors who are approved as providers of the particular product or service. The vendors should be shown to be qualified to provide quality products or services. A general approval of a vendor does not make sense as will be noted below. A combination of supplier assessment and material receiving acceptance activities should be used to meet this requirement. The company that provides excellent cleanroom maintenance services may not be the best vendor of instrument calibration services. Contract testing laboratories, like any other suppliers of services, should be assessed for their ability to properly perform particular tests. Consultants should be chosen for their documented ability to provide expertise in a particular area. All suppliers must be assessed, and if the manufacturer does not have sufficient personnel or facilities to conduct these assessments, consultants or third party certifications might be accepted for a short period of time. However, each supplier should eventually undergo direct assessment by the manufacturer. The assessment should evaluate the supplier on the basis of the supplier's compliance with standards such as the EN, ISO, or CFR; the supplier's performance history; and past provision of acceptable material.

Ultimately, this document must provide for some coordination of activities between the quality systems (see 21 CFR 820.5) and purchasing functions. This regulation brings certain purchasing functions under the mantle of the quality system, and it is important to define the interfaces between the two activities.

36. **Vendor Qualification.** The next document written to fulfill the requirements of 21 CFR 820.50 should establish the evaluation criteria and procedures that the manufacturer intends to use with different vendors. Most manufacturers use a graded approach that depends on the criticality of the product or service. A supplier that is already meeting CGMP or ISO standards can be given some credit for that status. The supplier of a key component of the device (patient contact or high potential for serious consequences from a malfunction) should be expected to provide a product that meets full quality requirements. Remember that the vendor of a component that will be used in further manufacturing activities may not be held to CGMP requirements under the Quality System regulations. At the same time, the manufacturer will want to verify the ability of the vendor to meet minimum quality requirements for the component that is being purchased. The vendor may need to be audited if testing or inspection alone will not be sufficient to establish the ability of the component to perform in a safe and efficacious manner. The manufacturer should expect such a supplier to have a quality system that meets the manufacturer's standards, and this should be established by quality audits of the supplier and checking the incoming product. Quality audits will be external audits as discussed in 21 CFR 820.22. If the supplier is a manufacturer of the item supplied, it would not be unreasonable to ask to review Statistical Process Control (SPC) charts covering the production of the purchased item. Especially if a long-term relationship is being planned, the purchaser should receive some evidence that the producer has a stable process that is operating within good control limits. All of these requirements should be written into the purchase contract between the supplier and the manufacturer. A clearly defined relationship defining the level and extent of control that the manufacturer will exercise over the supplier should be developed.

    Suppliers of less critical products or services could be qualified by sending questionnaires and performing less frequent quality audits. This could be combined with incoming raw material inspections to verify the ability of the supplier to consistently meet the manufacturer's specifications. Suppliers of services could be checked by sending a questionnaire, checking references, and reviewing training records. Evaluations of consultants are usually done by the evaluation of a resume and a personal interview. Allowances could be made for companies that maintain ISO registration or are, themselves, subject to periodic FDA or other regulatory inspections. If this is done, there must be a follow-up to verify the ISO registration or check for outstanding issues with the FDA. This information is available to the public and should be reviewed. A manufacturer should have good reasons for signing a contract with a company that is being prosecuted by the FDA or has a manager that was debarred by the FDA.

Even if the manufacturer conducts in-house quality control testing on all incoming material, it should still conduct some investigations to verify the ability of the supplier to furnish acceptable products. This is based on the old Quality Assurance principle that testing alone cannot prove "goodness." The manufacturing of the item must be done with the goal of producing acceptable product, so some manner of assessment needs to be done to verify that the supplier has an operating quality system.

The evaluation of suppliers should be coordinated with or even assigned to the unit that performs internal quality audits as required by 21 CFR 820.22. Experienced auditors can perform both external and internal evaluations of quality systems, and by including technically qualified guest auditors, evaluate the technical quality of the vendor's product. Many auditors work with preaudit questionnaires that can easily be modified to become product specific. Because they should already be familiar with the internal process requirements of the manufacturer, the auditors can evaluate the properties of the vendor's product, and judge its ability to meet the requirements of the manufacturer's processes. Also, if an auditing team already exists, they can often respond to emergency needs when the processing of a questionnaire requires too much time. The FDA has agreed not to review supplier audit reports during routine inspections as stated in 21 CFR 820.180(c). However they may require the manufacturer's management to provide a certification that the audit was performed and evaluated.

One problem with these assessments arises from distributors. In many cases, a part or component will be provided by a distributor who only serves as an intermediary between the actual producer of the part or component and the manufacturer. The purchase contract and specification, however, is between the manufacturer and distributor. In some cases, the distributor may be obtaining the item from several producers, all of whom produce to the same set of specifications but do not necessarily have equivalent quality systems. In other instances, the distributor may be reluctant to reveal the identity and location of the producer for fear that the manufacturer will eventually go directly to the producer, bypassing the distributor. These situations usually require a good amount of diplomacy, along with creative approaches, such as offering long-term contracts to the distributor and contracts requiring the use of only certain "cleared" producers for the manufacturer's products. Sometimes a little bit of investigation through catalogs and manufacturer's indices will allow an engineer or other technically qualified individual to determine the actual producer of the item without having to involve the distributor. Some producers will have contracts that allow them to sell only through particular distributors, and this is fine as long as a direct assessment can be made of the producer. In all of these situations, it is probably wise to assess both the producer and the distributor, since bad handling and storage practices on the part of the distributor may affect the quality of the part or component. If it is not possible to assess the real supplier, it will be necessary to rely on incoming raw material acceptance testing.

It is often useful to have a second vendor for a critical component or supply item. This is especially true of technically advanced products where the number of potential vendors is small, and the vendors themselves are small companies of uncertain future. The manufacturer may wish to qualify two vendors and divide orders between the two as a hedge against the loss of a vendor. This may not be possible or reasonable if there is a close relationship between the vendor and manufacturer as may arise in situations where a vendor specifically provides a product that meets the manufacturer's criteria. The requirements of a Just-in-Time or other, similar, system may also preclude the use of a second vendor. In these cases the manufacturer must develop a system for closely monitoring the business health and quality system of the vendor.

The reports resulting from these evaluations should be placed in special vendor files that will be available to purchasing and quality assurance personnel. All vendor evaluations should be placed in these files. If a vendor who failed an initial evaluation later submits an offer to supply the same or a different product, the individual conducting the new evaluation should be aware of the circumstances attending the earlier rejection. Also, the holding period for these documents should be defined as well as who has responsibility for maintaining the files.

37. **Manufacturer's Control.** This document will specify the extent and methods of control that the manufacturer will exercise over suppliers and the documentation of these activities. It should consider questions such as the following:

❖ What are the consequences if incoming lots of components fail the manufacturer's testing?
❖ What happens to the janitorial service if roaches infest a reagent preparation area?
❖ What happens to the purchasing commitment if the vendor fails future quality audits, refuses to take corrective actions requested by auditors, or the product repeatedly fails to meet the incoming quality standards?

The type of inspection to be conducted by the manufacturer should be spelled out, and the consequences of not meeting the requirements of the inspection stated. These considerations should be spelled out in the purchasing contract, so this document needs to become a part of the manufacturer's purchasing procedures. It might be useful to specify standard phrases or clauses that must be included in all of the manufacturer's purchasing contracts.

The agreement described for paragraph 21 CFR 820.50(b) below should also be included as a statement for the purchasing contract. It may seem simple to enter a statement requiring the vendor to inform the manufacturer of any changes in the product or service, but the consequences may be complex. In fact the purchaser may want to ask for a notification of any changes in the production methods or processing procedures, even if the vendor does not feel that there will be a change in the quality of the product being furnished. This need arises from the vendor's lack of knowledge regarding the manufacturer's device. The manufacturer should be more familiar with the properties of the device than the vendor of a part or service. Consequently, the manufacturer should be able to forecast the consequences of a change better than the vendor. Therefore, the manufacturer, not the vendor, should and does have the responsibility of deciding if a change might affect the quality of the manufacturer's product.

Once again a problem may arise with distributors. The distributor, itself, may not receive a notification of changes or may be in a poor position to force the producer to notify it of any changes. This is the reason for the "where possible" phrase in the regulation. The wise manufacturer will still want to try to obtain these agreements "where possible" because of the potentially serious consequences of a change that could affect the device's safety or efficacy. Again, some creative purchasing procedures could be employed to obtain these agreements.

An approach that is gaining favor and is covered by the ANSI/ISO/ASQC 9001 rules, is the inspection of product on the producer's premises. The manufacturer could send a representative to actually perform or participate in inspections during the production of the material. Also, if the producer is manufacturing under Statistical Process Control and has a process that is stable with control limits that meet the manufacturer's needs, the manufacturer could arrange to accept product that is produced under these conditions. Copies of control charts showing that the product was manufactured during a period when the process was stable and under control could be provided to the manufacturer. The manufacturer, in turn, would periodically audit the producer to verify the process control activities, and may periodically subject the product to inspection and testing to check the quality of the producer's activities. If this can be done in an efficient manner, it may provide the manufacturer with significant savings.

The use of contracted services is also an area of concern. In particular, the Quality Systems Manual contains a long discussion of the requirements for dealing with contract sterilizers. Basically, a contractor providing services must be treated as though it was providing a product, which the service is. If this principle is followed, the manufacturer should be able to devise a good quality approach for dealing with these contractors.

21 CFR 820.50(b) Purchasing Data. *Each manufacturer shall establish and maintain data that clearly describe or reference the specified requirements, including quality requirements, for purchased or otherwise received product and services. Purchasing documents shall include, where possible, an agreement that the suppliers, contractors, and consultants agree to notify the manufacturer of changes in the product or service so that manufacturers may determine whether the changes may affect the quality of a finished device. Purchasing data shall be approved in accordance with Sec. 820.40.*

38. **Purchasing Specifications.** The purchasing data document needs to require the establishment of specifications for purchased products and services. These purchase specifications should be the same as or include the product acceptance specifications. Designated files for the product specifications should be established and maintained and made accessible to purchasing, raw material quality control personnel, and the manufacturer's auditors (see 21 CFR 820.22), who should periodically check the vendor's compliance, or ability to comply, with the purchasing contract and specifications. Service specifications should be available to auditors or supervisors who are responsible for checking on the performance of contracted servicers, including consultants. To aid in the preparation of these specifications, templates or specific formats should be designed, especially since the documents may be used by several departments. The resulting specifications should then be incorporated directly into the purchasing contracts. In some companies, these specifications are attached to each purchase order to avoid confusion over exactly what is

being ordered. If useful, drawings or prints may be used in place of written purchasing specifications.

It is possible that the specifications or properties of an item are very well known and mere mention of the tradename is sufficient to establish the product specifications and quality of the product. However, even in these cases, the manufacturer should have at least an internal document listing the necessary product specifications. At a minimum, the internal document should list the specifications and tolerances that are necessary for the item to be used with the manufacturer's device. This document should also include test criteria with instructions to conduct occasional tests to verify that the product meets the manufacturer's needs. In the current business climate, it is foolish to expect that any product will be produced for a long time without any attempt to modify it to try to gain the last possible fraction of profit or production advantage.

The specifications should be based on requirements that were developed during the design process and should meet the requirements of the design input (see 21 CFR 820.30 (c)). Product specifications or supplied material specifications should address all properties of the component that will be important for the inclusion of the item in the product. The manufacturer must be sure to address all critical factors, even minor ones. Otherwise, the vendor may change that factor without warning. Quality specifications must be included. The vendor should be told what tolerances are expected and the methods by which the specifications will be monitored. For certain measurements, the vendor and manufacturer may want to come to an agreement on how measurements will be made so that common instruments or gauges may be designed and prepared.

Service specifications are important for maintaining continuity over time, especially when the service is multifaceted or where there are many possible ways that servicing may be performed. A contract laboratory that changes to procedures that were not a part of the license application or a janitorial service that sprays hallways with a pesticide that is not approved for use can create major problems. As with product specifications, the manufacturer must specify the dimensions of the service, including the permissible variations. The evaluation method that the manufacturer will use also must be specified.

The mechanism for the review and approval of these specifications must be defined, including the requirement for an approval date and signatures of the approvers. The approval date is important as a control of the currency of the document. In a large organization, the manner of the approval routing must be specified, as one may expect that different documents will need to be reviewed by personnel with knowledge in different areas. As part of this routing, it may be very useful to have the vendor included as a reviewer. It is very important to have the vendor aware of exactly what it is expected to supply before the presentation of a purchasing contract. It is also important to ensure that the vendor is not being asked to meet specifications beyond its capabilities. Contracts are often reviewed and signed by personnel who have only a hazy idea about the technical requirements that are being accepted. This can be especially true if the purchases are made through a distributor.

There should be a requirement for a periodic review and reissuance of these documents to allow for a periodic check to ensure that the specifications meet current needs. This process should involve a new review and approval by current personnel who are involved with the production of the device. The manufacturer needs to avoid the situation that arises when the vendor makes changes that are informally accepted by the manufacturer's personnel (a receiving clerk, for example), who fail to inform the rest of the company. This can happen when a telephone call describing a technically significant change is made to the manufacturer's purchasing agent, who verbally agrees to the change and fails to inform the rest of the organization or discuss the change with a technically qualified individual. A considerable amount of nonconforming product can be manufactured before the purchaser discovers the problem. Over a period of years, a large number of changes can accumulate before they are discovered during a vendor quality audit. Any changes in the product or service specifications should be reviewed and approved by the same route used with a new specification.

❋ Subpart F—Identification ❋ and Traceability

21 CFR 820.60 Identification

Each manufacturer shall establish and maintain procedures for identifying product during all stages of receipt, production, distribution, and installation to prevent mixups.

39. **Product Identification.** This document will establish a method to uniquely identify each batch, unit, or lot of raw material, manufacturing material, intermediate product, or finished product at all stages of the manufacturing and distribution processes. The general rule should be that, at any point where the device or its precursors "come to rest," they should have a highly visible label bearing a unique identifier and the acceptance status as required by 21 CFR 820.86. The label does not really need to state the acceptance status but the requirements of 21 CFR 820.86 need to be met and the efficient course would be to combine both requirements on the same label.

The document needs to define the form and color of the label and the information that will be included on the label. The method for generating the unique identification for each lot should also be specified, so that all of the company's products and intermediates will be subject to uniform identification procedures. Separate shipments of the same lot number should receive different identifiers, as the possibility exists that the material will be exposed to differing environmental conditions or handling procedures during shipment. This may mean that acceptance activities may need to be repeated on the same supplier's lot of material. The problem here is not the requirement for reassessing separate shipments of material, but with the bad planning that leads to the necessity for accepting multiple shipments of the same lot of material.

Note that 21 CFR 820.65 defines certain types of devices that are elsewhere known as critical devices. These types of devices must be assigned a unique identifier in the form of a control number. This control number should be used with the labeling described here. Remember that under the "where appropriate" provisions, it is not necessary to devise an elaborate label and control number system if the manufacturer only has one product.

The identifier should be attached to the outside of containers holding the product so that it is not necessary to open the container or refer to records to know what the contents are and where the contents are in the manufacturing process. With devices that exist as discrete units, the same could be done by placing the devices into an enclosed and locked mobile cage or by placing individual tags on the units. The document on identification should contain a statement requiring all processing documents to state the requirement for identification of the product at appropriate stages. In fact, the need for identification of the product at all stages should be a factor covered in the design development and planning in 21 CFR 820.30(b). This statement should also describe the means of affixing the identification. For instance, if the device itself cannot be labeled with a control number, it might be sealed in a container, which would then be labeled with the control number.

21 CFR 820.65 Traceability

Each manufacturer of a device that is intended for surgical implant into the body or to support or sustain life and whose failure to perform when properly used in accordance with instructions for use provided in the labeling can be reasonably expected to result in a significant injury to the user shall establish and maintain procedures for identifying with a control number each unit, lot or batch of finished devices and where appropriate components. The procedures shall facilitate corrective action. Such identification shall be documented in the DHR.

40. **Tracing System.** The traceability document should use any control numbers or identifiers generated in 21 CFR 820.60 (Identification) and create a requirement that this number or code be recorded on every device unit and every document related to the handling of the product. If necessary, this document should state where or when the number should be recorded, including a clear statement of how it is to be entered into the device history record. The idea here is that the control number

should allow the manufacturer to trace the history of the device back to its individual raw material components, and identify the personnel who were involved in its manufacturing. The components of the device should also be traceable, especially if an individual component may pose a safety or health hazard on its own, separate from the device. For example, the material used to make an implant needs to be tracked as well as the implant itself, especially in situations where one lot of component will be used to make more than one lot of product or where more than one lot of component is used in making one lot of devices. The distribution records that can be used for tracing must be available for inspection as given in 21 CFR 820.160.

Note that particular types of devices may have their own identification and traceability requirements different from those listed in this short paragraph of the CGMPs. Cardiac pacemakers are covered in 21 CFR 805, *In Vitro* Diagnostic devices in 21 CFR 809, and general tracking requirements are given for the devices listed in 21 CFR 821. The devices mentioned in 21 CFR 820.65 need to be tracked only as far as the initial consignee, while 21 CFR 821 requires tracking to the patient. The manufacturer should be aware of any specific requirements that may apply to a particular device. At a minimum, traceability will be required for the "critical devices" listed in the Federal Register of March 17, 1988, and for *In Vitro* Diagnostics (see 21 CFR 809.10(a)(9)). The FDA has stated that it will notify affected manufacturers directly if it should determine that a device is subject to traceability requirements. This is especially important to consider as there have been many critical devices that have become available since 1988, and CDRH is quite aware that the 1988 list is seriously outdated.

Finally, the whole issue of traceability must be addressed. If the manufacturer decides that traceability is not required for a device, the manufacturer should be prepared to show the results of risk analysis or other studies on the device and its components to justify this conclusion. This regulation requires the use of a control number with the devices that it describes, which suggests that it is not necessary to use control numbers under all circumstances or for all devices. This is true. However, this is an age when manufacturers of soda pop and candy bars use control numbers on their products. Medical devices almost by definition affect the public health, and all prudent manufacturers already use control numbers, at least internally, to allow for manufacturing and quality assurance activities. Rather than try to avoid the use of identification and traceability procedures, it is probably best for the manufacturer of any but the most innocuous device to proceed on the assumption that control numbers or identifiers should be used and have tracing methods put in place.

❦ Subpart G—Production ❦ and Process Controls

21 CFR 820.70 Production and Process Controls

21 CFR 820.70(a) General. Each manufacturer shall develop, conduct, control, and monitor production processes to ensure that a device conforms to its specifications. Where deviations from device specifications could occur as a result of the manufacturing process, the manufacturer shall establish and maintain process control procedures that describe any process controls necessary to ensure conformance to specifications. Where process controls are needed they shall include:

(1) *Documented instructions, standard operating procedures (SOPs), and methods that define and control the manner of production;*
(2) *Monitoring and control of process parameters and component and device characteristics during production;*
(3) *Compliance with specified reference standards or codes;*
(4) *The approval of processes and process equipment; and*
(5) *Criteria for workmanship which shall be expressed in documented standards or by means of identified and approved representative samples.*

41. **Run Sheets or Work Instructions.** A document is needed to require the preparation of specific operating instructions (sometimes known as run sheets or work instructions) for all processing steps. This document should require the following:

a. The creation of run sheets containing step-by-step instructions on how the device is to be made; including procedures for any subassemblies; information about when samples are to be taken for testing; information about when tests are to be run; spaces for recording the results of any in-process tests, especially those involved in go-no-go decisions; and the signatures or initials of the individuals who perform each step. This document should have been produced during the design transfer step (21 CFR 820.30(h)).

   i. The run sheets should contain instructions on the procedures to be followed in the event that there are test failures or that unusual events occur during processing. The run sheets should contain instructions on actions to take to monitor and control process parameters and product characteristics, as well as references to equipment preparation directions, and so on.

b. The standards or models to be used for comparison or the gauges to be used for checking should be specified. These should also include criteria for workmanship. Workmanship criteria may need to be specified in a separate document that covers things such as smoothing of cut surfaces, surface roughness criteria, paint uniformity, and so on.

c. The document that describes the preparation of the run sheets should refer to the standards or codes that the product must meet and also refer to any process control procedures relevant to the manufacturing of the particular device. The run sheets for particular segments of the production process should, in turn, refer to the applicable process control procedures, standards, or codes.

d. The run sheets may need to accommodate requirements arising from various regulations. Maintenance of processing equipment should be considered, along with any resulting necessity to temporarily remove an item from service for maintenance or recalibration. If in-process adjustments to equipment are needed, then the requirements of 21 CFR 820.70(g)(3) should be included. If the removal or limitation of manufacturing material is a concern, the requirements of 21 CFR 820.70(h) should be addressed. Also, any steps that require handling of components, intermediates, or finished product should be performed with the requirements of 21 CFR 820.140 in mind.

42. **Process Initiation.** While it may be expected that previous process validation activities will have resulted in an approved process that may be run at will, some firms may wish to create a document to control the actual initiation of the process. This approval to start or to initiate the process is often useful because it allows management to establish the readiness of the company to begin production. In many companies, this approval is accomplished via a computer based scheduling process, but others may wish to follow a checklist much like an airplane pilot's preflight checklist. For a start, the checklist should include a verification that the facility is ready for use. This would include items such as cleanliness, environmental controls, and "line clears." This type of approval to process can verify that the correct process has been set up, all needed facilities and material will be available at the right time and present in the proper quantities, all needed equipment is available in the proper condition, and appropriate personnel are available.

   A checklist-type of approval to process can be useful if the company is running multiple processes that may resemble or draw resources from each other; if the process is such that a "hold" cannot be tolerated because of unstable intermediate products; or if the company is resource strapped, it may be very important to establish the fact that everything really is in place and available. In these resource limited situations, it is good to have the process approved at the start of each run.

43. **Release of Process Equipment.** Approval of the process equipment is also important and related to the approval of the process. The difference is that the equipment should be approved for use regardless of whether or not the company approves the initiation of a process. The document that controls the approval of process equipment should specify procedures for identifying each significant item of equipment that will be used in processing. The document should note that each equipment item should have a document associated with it that contains the instructions for cleaning and storing the item

and instructions on how it is to be prepared for use in processing. If the item can be used in more than one process, the instructions should be specific for each process in which it could be employed. The criteria that must be met before the item can be released for use should be described, along with references to any tests that must be passed. This approval of equipment can be very important for equipment that must be sterile or that is used for producing different products under conditions where cross contamination must be prevented.

21 CFR 820.70(b) Production and Process Changes. *Each manufacturer shall establish and maintain procedures for changes to a specification, method, process, or procedure. Such changes shall be verified or where appropriate validated according to Sec. 820.75, before implementation, and these activities shall be documented. Changes shall be approved in accordance with Sec. 820.40.*

44. **Production Change Control.** Product and process changes should result in a change to the contents of a document. Consequently, the change should be handled through the same mechanism that was developed for handling document changes in 21 CFR 820.40 and described in Part I. It is critical to choose appropriate individuals to review the change. At a minimum, the design review team should be consulted along with the design development team, if necessary. Approval of the document change will constitute approval of the product or process change, and the distribution of the changed document to appropriate personnel will act as the mechanism to communicate the change. The need here is for a document to specify the handling of the changes through the document change control process as described in 21 CFR 820.40(b) and to require the attachment of a document describing the verification study or validation activity that validates or verifies the acceptability of the change (see 21 CFR 820.75). The document describing this study should accompany the request for the document change, and a policy statement should be issued to the effect that this type of document change shall not be accepted for processing without an accompanying acceptability document.

   An important step is to decide on the need for validation. The regulation states that validation is needed when verification in the form of testing and inspection are not sufficient to verify fully the results of the change. However if this is a design change, design verification and validation activities should be required.

Guidance is available on when changes need to be validated. The FDA has published "Guidelines on General Principles of Process Validation" and has stated that whenever variables may affect a process, the process must be validated. Sterilization, molding, and welding were given as examples of processes that must be validated.

To streamline the process, the manufacturer may wish to have the actual validation or verification studies filed separately from the document change requests. In this case, a standard summary sheet should be developed to provide summary information on the study and to accompany the document change request. The validation or verification study itself needs to be reviewed and accepted with an acceptance date and signatures of those approving the study. This responsibility will usually fall on the design review team.

21 CFR 820.70(c) Environmental Control. *Where environmental conditions could reasonably be expected to have an adverse effect on product quality, the manufacturer shall establish and maintain procedures to adequately control these environmental conditions. Environmental control system(s) shall be periodically inspected to verify that the system, including necessary equipment, is adequate and functioning properly. These activities shall be documented and reviewed.*

45. **Environmental Control.** The manufacturer should have a basic document describing the heating, ventilation, and air-conditioning (HVAC) system in the manufacturing and storage areas. This is done because of a basic need to have a reasonable environment in the manufacturing and storage areas, even if the device does not specifically require such an environment. Wide temperature swings, stagnant air, toxic fumes, or a dusty work environment are unpleasant for employees and may result in unpleasant regulatory actions (not necessarily from the FDA) directed toward the manufacturer. The basic document must establish a system for periodic (perhaps yearly) inspections and maintenance on the HVAC system. The document should specify what is to be inspected or checked (e.g., air flow rates

or ambient particulate matter) and what maintenance will be performed (e.g., oil the fans, change the air filters). The results of these inspections, checks, and maintenance should be summarized in a report, which should be reviewed by appropriate management with a sign-off to verify that the review took place in a timely manner. A mechanism should also be created for a periodic review of several of these records to see if the aging of equipment is leading toward a major problem in the performance of the HVAC system. The major review could be done annually, simultaneously with the review of the current year's report. It might be appropriate to review reports from the previous three years with the fourth year being the current report.

All of this becomes more critical if there are environmental factors that could affect the performance of the device. If factors such as temperature, humidity, or airborne particulate matter are critical, it may be necessary to continuously monitor these factors throughout the manufacturing and distribution process. Other factors, not normally considered as part of monitoring a HVAC system, may need to be monitored. For example, particle size distribution may be important if the device is sensitive to particles of a defined size, and the possibility of electrostatic discharges or fields may be important for computerized devices. In these cases the document should specify monitoring procedures and frequencies and also specify more frequent inspections and reviews (perhaps daily or weekly) to allow the manufacturer to provide a high level of assurance that the product could not have been adversely affected during processing and holding. The FDA may review these documents that cover the activities of the environmental control system.

The manufacturer may wish to obtain a copy of U.S. Federal Standard 209E covering the classification of cleanrooms and clean zones with regard to particle removal. When classifying and validating clean areas this is a very useful document which provides the manufacturer with a well regarded and well recognized standard to meet.

21 CFR 820.70(d) Personnel. *Each manufacturer shall establish and maintain requirements for health, cleanliness, personal practices, and clothing of personnel if contact between such personnel*

*and product or environment could reasonably be expected to have
an adverse effect on product quality. The manufacturer shall ensure
that maintenance and other personnel who are required to work
temporarily under special environmental conditions are appropriately trained or supervised by a trained individual.*

46. **Personnel Environmental Control.** The first part of the requirement in 21 CFR 820.70(d) will be one or more documents that
define manufacturing-related personnel practices. Exactly what
these practices are will depend on the product and the systems
used for its manufacture and the personnel employed at particular manufacturing stages. In most cases, manufacturing employees will be required to wear special clothing in the work area,
because street clothing alone is usually considered unsuitable
for biomedical work environments. Another standard procedure
is to require hand washing and the wearing of clean gloves, eye
protection, and closed-toe shoes in the work area. If particle
containment is of concern, the use of cosmetics is usually restricted. Particle-free clothing or specially prepared garments are
usually employed along with hair and beard covers, and over-
shoes. Toilet facilities should be adequate for the number of employees in a shift.

In aseptic processing areas, a surgical face mask would be
added to the preceding list, and the garments would be sterile.
Jewelry should not be worn into these areas, since it is almost
impossible to clean jewelry, and it has a tendency to snag or
tear garments and gloves. In addition, coughing or sneezing employees should be excluded from the work area. Surgical masks,
even very good ones, usually cannot contain or process the air
expelled in a cough or sneeze. If the sterility of the device (including freedom from viruses) is critical, employees who report
to work while ill should be excluded from the manufacturing
area and temporarily assigned to other duties.

While these procedures are primarily designed to protect
the product from the personnel, it may be necessary to protect
the personnel from the work environment. Special practices
may need to be instituted. Garments or protective gear that are
dictated by processing methods should be compatible with the
needs mentioned in the previous paragraphs. For instance, in a

noisy aseptic processing area, hearing protection should be of a type that can be worn under the hair covering. Personnel who handle radioactive or highly carcinogenic substances should wear appropriate protective garments, and have decontamination facilities available.

Finally, one should remember that guests (auditors and/or inspectors!) may need to enter the work areas as well as new employees, so generic garments and related items should be available for these individuals. Also, it is a common practice to have posted instructions (sometimes with pictures) to instruct and remind employees of proper procedures to follow when gowning before entering controlled areas. All of these procedures and even the wording of the posters should be included in the document that specifies these practices. Depending on the local employee population, bilingual or multilingual posters may be needed. The employees should be trained to understand the need for sanitation and personal cleanliness as well as the procedures for meeting specific environmental requirements. This training should be documented.

47. **Personnel Training.** The second document needed for this part of the CGMP is one that requires the training of all production and processing employees in the proper performance of their jobs and in the practices noted above. Personal hygiene and contamination awareness training may need to be performed. This document should specifically require the training of employees who may need to work temporarily under special environmental conditions and provide for an exemption if the work will be performed under the supervision of a trained individual. This document should be compatible with the requirements of 21 CFR 820.25(b) and should state that all training of production personnel shall be documented and records will be placed in personnel training files. Without being too specific, this document should describe the training to be provided and the mechanism for documenting and recording the training. It should also define what training is required for an employee to be considered a "trained individual."

One important consideration that needs to go along with the training concept is the need for functional literacy. It is unfortunately common to encounter an employee (usually a new one) who is unable to read and understand the documents related to that employee's work functions. Even among college graduates, one may encounter personnel who can read words but cannot understand their meaning in the context of the work to be done. For this reason, training may need to be done at what appears to be a very low educational level. The manufacturer should never assume that any employee can take a document and read and understand it without specific training in its execution. Monumental blunders have occurred, and the cost saving from preventing just one of these blunders can often justify a whole training program.

21 CFR 820.70(e) Contamination Control. *Each manufacturer shall establish and maintain procedures to prevent contamination of equipment or product by substances that could reasonably be expected to have an adverse effect on product quality.*

21 CFR 820.70(f) Buildings. *Buildings shall be of suitable design and contain sufficient space to perform necessary operations, prevent mixups, and assure orderly handling.*

The regulations regarding buildings and contamination control are of the type that seem obvious but must be stated to ensure completeness. The rational person will do these things as a matter of course, but if they are not stated, there are those who will attempt to excuse their mistakes by saying, "Well it didn't say we *had* to do it." Consequently, it would appear that it is not necessary to have separate documents to describe the application of these regulations. Contamination control should be effectively handled in documents covering the environment (21 CFR 820.70 (c)), production and process instructions (21 CFR 820.70(a)), handling (21 CFR 820.140), storage (21 CFR 820.150), distribution (21 CFR 820.160), and installation (21 CFR 820.170). Note that the regulation covers both equipment and product. There is an implication that the design of the equipment should allow for easy maintenance, cleaning or prevention of contamination (21 CFR 820.70(g)). Factors related to buildings should be covered in general planning for the manufacturing facilities, and checked during any facility validation studies. Basically the buildings must be adequate for their intended uses.

Contaminants resulting from the application of rodenticides, fungicides or insecticides must be minimized. These agents should meet Federal environmental requirements and also the requirements for use in food establishments. They should never be employed in critical manufacturing areas. The manufacturer should depend on general housekeeping practices to prevent the entry of foreign organisms into the manufacturing areas. Even with these precautions, substances such as insecticides may be carried into work areas on employee clothing or skin. The manufacturer's employees must maintain an awareness of the agents used by any contracted exterminator, and have the information on file for review. In fact this review of the agents to be used by an exterminator should be conducted as a part of the vendor approval process (21 CFR 820.50(a)).

On the subject of environmental and contamination control, it appears that the use of barriers and isolator technology is gaining favor for situations where maximum cleanliness and sterility are important. The manufacturer may wish to investigate these technologies and at least ensure that documents and licenses are prepared in such a way that a switch to these technologies may occur with a minimum of problems. With many devices, there will be additional requirements for environmental conditions that meet semiconductor industry requirements in addition to medical device industry requirements. The incorporation of logic circuits in devices created these requirements. Medical device manufacturers must ensure environmental conditions that are good for the semiconductor portion of the devices.

21 CFR 820.70(g) Equipment. *Each manufacturer shall ensure that all equipment used in the manufacturing process meets specified requirements and is appropriately designed, constructed, placed, and installed to facilitate maintenance, adjustment, cleaning, and use.*

48. **Equipment Capability.** The first part of 21 CFR 820.70(g) will be met by a combination of design output (21 CFR 820.30 (d)) and purchasing controls (21 CFR 820.50(a)), because the design output should give the equipment capabilities that must be present to produce a product that will satisfy the design requirements. The purchasing process should transmit these equipment capability requirements as part of the purchasing specifications for the equipment. If the equipment is not purchased, but made by an internal group, the internal contract for producing the equipment should transmit this information to the producer

group. The company should then develop a document that gives the requirement for equipment design review, equipment design acceptance, and finished equipment acceptance by the department or group that will use the equipment.

49. **Equipment Qualification Procedures.** The second document needed to satisfy 21 CFR 820.70(g) is one that will require the use of equipment qualification procedures. This consists of IQ (installation qualification), OQ (operating qualification), and PQ (process qualification). In other words, is the equipment installed properly and does it meet the supplier's specifications as installed (IQ); does it operate as specified by the supplier and required by the purchasing group (OQ); and, finally, does the equipment perform as required during actual processing (PQ)? The document should require consideration of the equipment design, construction, placement, installation, maintenance, and cleaning in addition to actual equipment use as factors in the qualification studies. This second document should give a format for these studies and a format for the qualification reports. These qualification reports should be placed in the file for the equipment item. These equipment qualification activities should be extended to the equipment mentioned in 21 CFR 820.72.

The need for periodic requalification should also be addressed. The idea is to ensure the ability of the equipment to perform properly as long as it is in use. The need for requalification could arise when routine maintenance was no longer sufficient and a major refurbishing was required, or after a major breakdown where one or more major parts had to be replaced. Another situation that is more common would be the gradual accumulation of small defects due to wear and tear that eventually lead to equipment that cannot be maintained in its qualified state for reasonable lengths of time.

50. **Equipment Files.** For reasons that go beyond the regulation under consideration here, the manufacturer should develop a set of equipment files. These files should document the history and use of each critical item of equipment. (The term *critical item* refers to equipment whose operations or properties could affect the quality of the finished device.) The file should contain copies of the design requirements for the item, the equipment

design review and approval, the purchasing specifications, the supplier's specifications, the qualification studies, the releases and approvals for use as given for 21 CFR 820.70(a)(4), reports of maintenance activities from 21 CFR 820.70(g)(1), any calibration reports, and a record of the final disposition of the item if it is no longer used. The manufacturer may have other documents to include in this file. Also, each critical equipment item should have a unique control number that is specific to each item. This number should be affixed to the item, and should be used to facilitate cross referencing especially if the manufacturer has an electronic tracking system. Maintenance activities specified in 21 CFR 820.72 should follow a similar procedure. The file should be retained as specified in 21 CFR 820.180(b) using the dating of the last batch or lot manufactured using the item.

21 CFR 820.70(g)(1) Maintenance Schedule. *Each manufacturer shall establish and maintain schedules for the adjustment, cleaning, and other maintenance of equipment to ensure that manufacturing specifications are met. Maintenance activities, including the date and individual(s) performing the maintenance activities, shall be documented.*

51. **Maintenance Schedule.** The requirements for the maintenance schedule document are clear from the regulation. It might be easiest to specify a maintenance summary sheet that would contain the required information. In addition to the information required by the regulation, it would be useful to add the following:

    ❖ The date for which the maintenance activity was scheduled.
    ❖ A short summary of what activities were performed.
    ❖ Any unusual conditions or special observations.
    ❖ The date of completion of the activity.
    ❖ The signature of the person who performed the maintenance.

    A maintenance schedule needs to be posted near the equipment or otherwise be made readily available to the user personnel. The schedule might be a part of a "work calendar" that might be maintained on a computer or work station that the equipment operators are required to consult at the beginning of a shift.

21 CFR 820.70(g)(2) Inspection. Each manufacturer shall conduct periodic inspections in accordance with established procedures to ensure adherence to applicable equipment maintenance schedules. The inspections, including the date and individual(s) conducting the inspections, shall be documented.

52. **Maintenance Inspection.** These inspections could be conducted as a part of the internal auditing process noted in 21 CFR 820.22. The document required here is a specification or template for a short form that will be completed by the auditor or internal inspector. The short form will contain the information required above and also record the audit report date and audit control number for cross-referencing purposes. If the manufacturer prefers to use inspectors from the manufacturing group, this is fine as long as the document that controls these activities defines the procedures to be used and provides directions for the completion of the inspection forms.

21 CFR 820.70(g)(3) Adjustment. Each manufacturer shall ensure that any inherent limitations or allowable tolerances are visibly posted on or near equipment requiring periodic adjustments or are readily available to personnel performing these adjustments.

53. **Control of Adjustments.** In most instances, the adjustment requirement is met by using a label that is placed on the equipment in such a way that anyone attempting to make an adjustment must see the label. If it is not possible to label the equipment in this manner, a summary sheet with a prominent heading should be posted nearby or at the operator's desk or included in the SOP that must be used when performing the adjustment. The label or summary sheet should contain the information required above, the date of the last adjustment, and the date of the next adjustment with the initials of the person who performed the last adjustment. Clearly, this means that the label or sheet will need to be replaced periodically or after each adjustment. An original copy of the label or summary sheet should be placed in the equipment file mentioned earlier under 21 CFR 820.70(g). If the need for adjustments is relatively infrequent, it could be combined with the maintenance activities noted in 21 CFR 820.70(g)(1) and the activity recorded in the maintenance report.

If the adjustment must be made fairly frequently, an SOP for the adjustment along with a log book recording the time, date, and initials of the adjuster should be used. The SOP should be available at or close to the work station and clearly state the intervals between adjustments. Also, if possible, a prominent sign or label stating the need for adjustments at given intervals should be affixed to the equipment in a location clearly visible to the operator. The log book or sheet, when filled, should be placed in the equipment file for that item. If the adjustment is of the type that must be made during a manufacturing run, the requirements for the adjustment could be written into the production run sheets described in 21 CFR 820.70(a). Most manufacturers will have equipment requiring adjustments at various intervals, so all methods described above might be in use at the same time.

The document needed to fulfill 21 CFR 820.70(g)(3) will describe the format or template for the label, summary sheet, or log book, ensuring that they accommodate the requirements mentioned above. If the company does not have much equipment, the requirements for each item might be given in this single document. Otherwise, this document should specify the contents and format of an "equipment adjustment SOP" that would be specific to each equipment item. The SOP will say what adjustments need to be made, what the tolerances or limitations are, the intervals between adjustments, and how the adjustment is to be verified and recorded.

21 CFR 820.70(h) Manufacturing Material. *Where a manufacturing material could reasonably be expected to have an adverse effect on product quality, the manufacturer shall establish and maintain procedures for the use and removal of such manufacturing material to ensure that it is removed or limited to an amount that does not adversely affect the device's quality. The removal or reduction of such manufacturing material shall be documented.*

21 CFR 820.3(p) Manufacturing material *means any material or substance used in, or used to facilitate, a manufacturing process, a concomitant constituent, or a by product constituent produced during the manufacturing process, which is present in or on the finished device as a residue or impurity not by design or intent of the manufacturer.*

The regulation regarding manufacturing material does not appear to create a need for a separate document or file. First of all, it must be considered only if there is a need to remove or limit excess manufacturing material or undesirable manufacturing by products. If the need exists, the first action will be to include activities in the manufacturing process to remove or limit excess manufacturing material. These activities should be included in the procedures specified in the run sheets described in 21 CFR 820.70(a). The second action needed here would be to include inspection or testing activities to verify the removal or limitation of the manufacturing material. These activities could be added to the documents specifying acceptance activities under 21 CFR 820.80(c) and (d).

Note that the term *manufacturing materials* is used as part of the definition of "product" in 21 CFR 820.3(r). Therefore manufacturing material needs to be treated like any other component if it is obtained and added to the system like a raw material. In addition, the terms *other byproducts of the manufacturing process* and *naturally occurring substance* have been combined to result in a statement under this regulation, that if a device utilizes natural rubber latex as a component, the allergenic proteins in the latex should be removed or reduced. This process could be described in a preparation run sheet or in a raw material product specification. Note also that the lubricating oil used with a machine may constitute a manufacturing material if it is transmitted to the device. A procedure would need to be developed to remove or limit the amount of this oil.

21 CFR 820.70(i) Automated Processes. *When computers or automated data processing systems are used as part of production or the quality system, the manufacturer shall validate computer software for its intended use according to an established protocol. All software changes shall be validated before approval and issuance. These validation activities and results shall be documented.*

54. **Software Validation Studies.** These activities should be coordinated with the activities described in document 26 (21 CFR 820.30(g)). Even small programs written for programmable calculators or built into instruments must be validated. All software used in data processing must be validated, whether it is used in designing, manufacturing, distributing, tracking, documentation, or quality systems. All changes to existing programs should

also be validated before introduction into general use following the principles given for 21 CFR 820.70(b). The validation should involve a review of the program code to verify the ability of the software to perform in the manner expected without introducing spurious or unnecessary events. If the software is obtained from a second party who does not wish to reveal the program code to the user, it may be necessary to create a provision for obtaining a review by a third party acceptable to the second party, who would execute a confidentiality agreement with the second party. This third party might be a consultant, who would write a validation report for submission to the manufacturer without revealing the program code. A less costly procedure, when this is acceptable to CDRH, is to use black box testing.

In black box testing, the software is probed by entering a variety of data and reviewing the output. A common situation here would be the case of a calculator that contains a built-in statistics package. A variety of data would be entered and the results of the calculations would be recorded. The results would then be compared to the results of manual calculations or calculations performed by a well-known software package. Validity would be established by showing that the calculator program generated the same results. The system must be probed with a wide range of data, including extreme and ridiculous inputs. The idea is to guard against situations where a glitch or spurious input nonetheless produces a result that appears rational.

The second step in the validation will be to introduce data into the system to determine its ability to correctly process the data and produce a good result. This is similar to the black box testing mentioned above but does not need to be as extensive, if the code has been verified. In most cases, these data will be derived from earlier work where pocket calculators or pencil and paper were used to calculate the correct result. Older textbooks with solved problems are often a convenient source of these data. The program must be challenged with aberrant data as well. Numbers at the extremes, words instead of numbers, and vice versa should be entered into the program to see if there is any possibility for obtaining apparently normal results from abnormal data. Although this is a different situation from the one that arises when software is used to program and operate the manufacturer's device, the need for design review and validation is the same, and similar procedures must be adopted.

The validation procedures discussed above are for use with smaller programs that are not widely distributed or are written locally. The document required here should describe the validation protocol that will be employed and the general format for the validation study report. The validation reports should be filed with the documents establishing the software system, except for reports on equipment related software, which should be placed in the equipment file. Validations of data processing software should be filed with the procedure that requires the data processing. Software changes should be subjected to change control and validation like any other documentation change, with the validation report required as a supporting document before the change can be approved.

In the case of large and complex programs, such as an information management system or a resource planning and scheduling system, it is usually best to employ a consulting firm to perform the validation, unless the manufacturer has a large and highly skilled computer services group or unless the supplier will work with the manufacturer to validate the software package after installation. Software validations are different from regular work and time consuming to the point where they can seriously disrupt the operations of an internal computer services group. A second problem arises from the fact that the programmers or other computer people within the company are often unfamiliar with the manufacturing operations or quality systems of the company and may have difficulty in designing appropriate validation studies. A correctly chosen consulting firm may be more familiar with the needs of the manufacturer.

It is usually not necessary to review the program code for widely distributed and well-known software packages. These are generally the better known word processors, spreadsheets, databases, or statistical software packages. The general assumption is that such software will be studied by many different groups; and bugs, glitches, and other assorted problems associated with the software will become well known through user groups and other publication mechanisms. Of course this assumes that user personnel will take the steps necessary to become informed users of the software.

It is still necessary to prove that the software is suitable for its intended use. This is especially true in the case of programs such as spreadsheets, where there are many functions or macros that may be employed in various combinations to make custom subroutines to handle particular needs. These applications need to be validated to show that the software is capable of performing its intended function.

In the Quality System Manual, CDRH provided references to guidance documents on software validation. These were: "Application of the Medical Device GMP's to Computerized Devices and Manufacturing Processes," and "Reviewer Guidance for Computer Controlled Medical Devices Undergoing 510(k) Review." Both of these are available from CDRH. Other relevant guidance documents listed were Military Specification MIL-S-52779A and the "Standard for Software Quality Assurance Plan" (IEEE Std 730-1984).

21 CFR 820.72 Inspection, Measuring, and Test Equipment

21 CFR 820.72(a) Control of Inspection, Measuring, and Test Equipment. Each manufacturer shall ensure that all inspection, measuring, and test equipment, including mechanical, automated, or electronic inspection and test equipment, is suitable for its intended purposes and is capable of producing valid results. Each manufacturer shall establish and maintain procedures to ensure that equipment is routinely calibrated, inspected, checked, and maintained. The procedures shall include provisions for handling, preservation, and storage of equipment, so that its accuracy and fitness for use are maintained. These activities shall be documented.

55. **Metrology Department.** In many, if not most, companies the process of routinely calibrating, inspecting, checking, and maintaining testing equipment is the responsibility of the metrology department. The first document that is needed establishes the department, assigns responsibilities for its operations, and defines

the scope of its function. It is not necessary to create a completely separate department. The function of the metrology department is often performed within the Plant Engineering or Quality Assurance departments. Remember that this function covers all inspection, measuring, and test equipment regardless of physical location. All laboratory equipment and environmental monitoring equipment that perform these functions need to be covered by the metrology system. The employees engaged in performing these functions need to be identified and trained in metrology and that training should be documented. The document that establishes the function should also describe a secondary set of documents that will describe the procedures for the calibration, checking and storage of equipment. These documents should also refer to activities relative to the "test software" that are employed with the "automated or electronic inspection and test equipment."

56. **Maintenance SOPs.** For each item or group of inspection, measuring, or test equipment there should be a maintenance SOP similar to the ones developed for production equipment in 21 CFR 820.70(g). This will refer specifically to the maintenance, handling, preservation and storage requirements of the inspection, measuring, or test equipment and not general equipment maintenance. The SOP should first specify the maintenance activities that will be needed, the intervals between the maintenance activities, the responsibility for the maintenance, and provisions for verifying that the maintenance occurred. Conditions under which the act of maintenance should lead to a calibration check should be specified. It is important to ensure that the maintenance does not result in instruments that have been inadvertently adjusted. In other words the act of maintenance results in adjusting the instrument settings. If this occurs, a recalibration should be performed as a part of the maintenance. Procedures for verifying the performance of software, after maintenance activities, should be specified, especially if there is the possibility that maintenance could result in the input of a false datum or a change in the programming.

Finally, it should be noted that for equipment that is extremely sensitive or delicate or is operating in an extreme environment, some validation may be required to show that the procedures for verifying that the maintenance activities are truly effective in maintaining the accuracy or fitness-for-use of the equipment are, themselves, valid. If equipment is constantly requiring re-calibration, or maintenance, the procedures for maintaining, handling, preserving, and storing the equipment to maintain accuracy or fitness-for-use should be questioned.

57. **Equipment Qualification.** The next document for 21 CFR 820.72(a) should establish procedures for qualifying the inspection, measuring, and test equipment as they are received by the company or put into place for their operation. These activities are often known as installation qualification (IQ) and operational qualification (OQ), and they are really the same as the corresponding activities normally conducted on production equipment (see 21 CFR 820.70 (g)). IQ is a verification that the instrument or equipment is capable of meeting the purchase specifications after it is installed at the company in its working location. OQ then shows that the equipment is capable of doing the job for which it was obtained. Under certain circumstances, that are usually obvious to the worker, IQ and OQ could be combined into a single procedure. Remember that the instrument must do its job under the full range of environmental and manufacturing conditions. As much as possible, these qualification studies should be performed with the equipment installed in its actual place of operation. Many instruments work perfectly well on a table in the receiving dock and then fail on the laboratory bench or on the production line.

As with any important equipment, each item should have a control number assigned to it so that it may be readily distinguished from other, similar items. For instance, each thermometer should have a unique control number, as should each gauge or template. Do not rely on vendor's serial numbers on the equipment because it is quite possible to have two distinctly different items with the same serial number, since the serial numbers are controlled by the individual producers. This control document should specify the format for the control numbers and assign the responsibility for generating and assigning the numbers. This is very important, as the company needs to have an unambiguous method to trace the history of important test and measuring equipment.

21 CFR 820.72(b) Calibration. *Calibration procedures shall include specific directions and limits for accuracy and precision. When accuracy and precision limits are not met, there shall be provisions for remedial action to reestablish the limits and to evaluate whether there was any adverse effect on the device's quality. These activities shall be documented.*

21 CFR 820.72(b)(1) Calibration Standards. *Calibration standards used for inspection, measuring, and test equipment shall be traceable to national or international standards. If national or international standards are not practical or available, the manufacturer shall use an independent reproducible standard. If no applicable standard exists, the manufacturer shall establish and maintain an in-house standard.*

58. **Calibration SOPs.** This document for 21 CFR 820.72(b) should establish the schedule for routine calibrations and classify the equipment if different classes will be on different schedules. Each type of instrument or equipment item should have its own protocol for calibration, inspection, checking, or maintenance; therefore this document should establish a template for the preparation of these protocols and a record form for documenting the calibration activity (see 21 CFR 820.72(b)(2)). In addition, the responsibility for maintaining the records, and the location of the records should be specified. This will create a set of calibration or metrology records. Each record will be specific for each item of measuring equipment and generated each time an instrument or equipment item is worked upon. Copies of these records should be held with the other records pertaining to the item in the equipment files created to meet the needs of 21 CFR 820.70 (g).

   The protocols (calibration SOPs) that give the procedures for calibrating, inspecting, checking, and maintaining each piece of equipment or, if possible, class of equipment (thermometers, for example), must include the information required in paragraphs 21 CFR 820.72(a) and (b). The protocol should create a summary sheet for each item that will contain the basic results of the calibration activity, the date performed, the date for the next calibration, and the signature of the individual responsible for the current calibration. It may be necessary to prepare a separate document to describe and establish the calibration standard, especially if it is an in-house standard. Also, if external laboratories or service groups are employed to perform the calibrations, it is important to verify the traceability of their calibration standards and to verify their qualifications to perform the calibration activities. Vendors of these services must be qualified like any other supplier to the manufacturer (see 21 CFR 820.50 (a)). This may require a direct audit by the individuals who perform audits under 21 CFR 820.22.

The calibration SOP should contain accuracy and precision specifications that must be met by the equipment after each recalibration. Directions for remedial action should be given in the event that the requirements for precision and accuracy cannot be met. The SOP should contain specific directions on how the accuracy and precision are to be measured for each item or each type of equipment. If the instrument makes measurements over a wide range, its precision and accuracy at the extremes of the range should be checked. Statistical methods used for establishing precision and accuracy should correspond to those in 21 CFR 820.250(a).

21 CFR 820.72(b)(2) Calibration records. *The equipment identification, calibration dates, the individual performing each calibration, and the next calibration date shall be documented. These records shall be displayed on or near each piece of equipment or shall be readily available to the personnel using such equipment and to the individuals responsible for calibrating the equipment.*

59. **Calibration Notification.** The requirements of 21 CFR 820.72(b)(2) are often met by placing a calibration sticker on the equipment. This sticker will contain the required information, including the control number of the item, and should be placed in a location that is easily visible to the operator. The document needed here should describe the use of these stickers, specify the information required on each sticker, and describe the general format of the sticker. The point is to prevent the use of an item that is overdue for its calibration or, worse, not calibrated.

The actual record of the calibration may be a single sheet kept in a log book that is conveniently located for the operator. The format for each sheet should be specified in each calibration SOP, and a copy of it along with a copy of the sticker being used should be placed in the equipment file for the particular item.

If a sticker cannot be used, the calibration requirements should be written into the operator instructions, especially the run sheets or daily work instructions, so that they are obvious to the operator. Individuals responsible for performing the calibrations could be reminded through the use of "tickler files." The preferred method here calls for the use of scheduling software whose display must be reviewed daily by the operator and individual responsible for the calibration.

21 CFR 820.75 Process Validation

21 CFR 820.75(a) Process Validation. Where the results of a process cannot be fully verified by subsequent inspection and test, the process shall be validated with a high degree of assurance and approved according to established procedures. The validation activities and results, including the date and signature of the individual(s) approving the validation and where appropriate the major equipment validated, shall be documented.

21 CFR 820.3(z)(1) Process Validation *means establishing by objective evidence that a process consistently produces a result or product meeting its predetermined specifications.*

60. **Process Validation.** This document needs to establish the procedures for process validation and the records, including equipment validations, that will be generated by the validation activities. The validation study will be basically aimed at demonstrating, in a verifiable way, that the process performs as expected and within the acceptable range of its parameters. It should also state the need for periodic revalidations because all processes drift over time with changes in personnel, material suppliers, equipment, and environment. The frequency of revalidation should be related to the importance of the process and its stability. If the process was important enough to validate, it is important enough to be maintained in a validated state. Most firms will have several processes that must be kept in a validated

state, and this document needs to describe general procedures applicable to all process validations. The criteria for a successful validation must be specified. One of the primary requirements will be the validation of supporting processes for the process validation. For instance, the process validation study should use assays and cleaning methods that are themselves validated. How can the validation study be valid if it is not based on validated procedures? This usually means that a statistician or quality engineer should be employed to design sampling procedures and aid in setting specifications. The range of the acceptance specifications is usually related to the criticality of the process and its stability. The first process validation study should be performed during the design verification and validation studies under 21 CFR 820.30(f) and (g), so that manufacturing will start with a process that is at least partially validated. Note that these process validations are ongoing activities and are only a part of the validations required to satisfy 21 CFR 820.30(g).

In the preamble to the CGMP regulations, the FDA has stated that all processes need some amount of qualification, verification, or validation, and manufacturers should not depend solely on inspection and testing to show that processes are adequate for their intended use. Examples of processes that require validation are sterilization, aseptic processing, injection molding, and welding.

It is often confusing to know what processes or processing steps require validation. The regulation states that one should consider situations where the results cannot be fully verified by subsequent inspection and test. A good example of this is sterility. If a sterilization step is used in the process, the only way to fully verify the sterilization is to test each unit that was sterilized, but this is highly impractical, so sterilization validation is normally done. In the case of cleaning, it is usually impractical to check the cleaning process before the item is used, so cleaning validations are also done as a matter of routine. Conversely, with certain types of injection molding processes, the operator checks the product or periodically samples the products to verify that the process is operating properly within a specified tolerance range. Another situation is when a solution undergoes dilution and an aliquot is taken for assay. Since the aliquot is representative of the whole volume of the solution, the assay will suffice for the whole volume. Both of these processes do not need to be validated as there are good procedures for verifying the result of the processing step.

A validation protocol needs to be written before the study is attempted, and its format should be specified in this document. To prove the consistency of the process, process validations usually require the study of three successive production runs. If there are validation studies that will be performed routinely and fairly frequently, standard protocols could be written for each type of study. A mechanism for the review and approval of the validation protocol needs to be specified, along with any notifications that may need to be given. For instance, it may be necessary to have the use of an autoclave or a filling line scheduled into an available time slot or certain equipment may need to be validated and scheduled for use before a validation study can be performed. Even routine validations need to be planned, and the planning needs to be approved.

In the Quality System Manual, the FDA gave the following as the basic elements for the purpose of a process validation:

❖ Establish that the processing equipment has the capability of operating within required parameters;
❖ Demonstrate that controlling, monitoring, and/or measuring equipment and instrumentation are capable of operating within the parameters prescribed for the processing equipment;
❖ Perform replicate cycles (runs) representing the required operational range of the equipment to demonstrate that the processes have been operated within the prescribed parameters for the process and that the output or product consistently meets predetermined specifications for quality and function; and
❖ Monitor the validated process during routine operation. As needed, requalify and recertify the equipment.

The elements that go into a process validation should be:

❖ Installation and Operational Qualification of processing equipment. This is to show that the process validation will be performed with equipment that is functioning properly.
❖ Assay or measurement method validations. These are needed to show that any assays or measurements made will meet acceptable standards for accuracy and precision.
❖ Environmental monitoring to assure that the manufacturing environment meets appropriate standards.
❖ Process Performance Qualification, which is often thought of as the only part of a process validation, needs to show that a product meeting specifications can be produced consistently when the process is operating within the specified limits. Note that there is a requirement to show the stability or reproducibility of the process, and this is done by validating three consecutive manufacturing runs.
❖ Product Performance Qualification may be combined with the design validation activities of 21 CFR 820.30(g). The devices produced during the product performance qualification may be checked to demonstrate conformance with manufacturing criteria and user needs.

In recent years there has been a trend for larger companies to form validation departments and have these groups actually perform the validations. In some cases such as sterilization this is understandable as the knowledge needed for a proper validation can be quite extensive or highly specific. The problem is that the validation study should reflect actual operating conditions, or a close surrogate. This will not happen when the study is done by a group that is specially picked for their knowledge of validation procedures or with a group of highly trained production workers who specialize in only performing validation studies. Ideally, the validation study should be performed by the actual workers who will run the process for the manufacturer. If a validation department must be formed, they should be QA/QC specialists in validations who will review validation study protocols and advise in their preparation and performance, but not actively participate in the work.

Validation studies of all types are usually expensive and often disruptive to normal operations, since the validations need to be conducted under actual operating conditions or under conditions that very closely mimic actual manufacturing conditions. Consequently, it is important to plan the activity beforehand to ensure a good, acceptable study that yields a maximum of usable data for the costs incurred. Also, the criteria for acceptance of the process need to be specified before the process is studied. Setting specifications after the study is completed implies that the manufacturer has no quality standards and is willing to accept whatever is found regardless of how bad or incorrect it may be or even if it is the result of sloppy or incompetent work.

The validation protocol and the study results should be placed in the DHF, while the procedures and actual manufacturing records for the runs used in the study should become a part of the DMR.

21 CFR 820.75(b) Monitoring and Control. *Each manufacturer shall establish and maintain procedures for monitoring and control of process parameters for validated processes to ensure that the specified requirements continue to be met.*

21 CFR 820.75(b)(1) *Each manufacturer shall ensure that validated processes are performed by qualified individual(s).*

21 CFR 820.75(b)(2) *For validated processes, the monitoring and control methods and data, the date performed, and, where appropriate, the individual(s) performing the process or the major equipment used shall be documented.*

21 CFR 820.75(c) Changes. *When changes or process deviations occur, the manufacturer shall review and evaluate the process and perform revalidation where appropriate. These activities shall be documented.*

A separate document is probably not needed to satisfy these regulations. Paragraphs 21 CFR 820.75(b) and (c) appear to be clear in their requirements, and these requirements should be included in the run sheets and documentation required under 21 CFR 820.75(a). The requirements of 21 CFR 820.75(b) are important in that most processes operate within a range of acceptable conditions. It is rare to find processes where parameters are set to a single, invariant value. As a result the manufacturer needs to know if a good, acceptable product will still be produced if the process operates at the extremes of the allowable ranges. In many studies the effects of going to the extremes of single ranges are given, but the manufacturer needs to know what will happen if all or most of the parameters should go to the extremes of their ranges. One of the problems here is that many companies evaluate a process at its extremes by making one run with all parameters set at their maxima and then making a second run with all parameters set at their minima. This is somewhat naive as some problems may not arise unless certain parameters are at their maxima, others at their minima, and others set in the center of their range. A process validation using a matrixed experimental design will go far to provide useful data to cover these situations. Training in the Design of Experiments (DOE) should be mandatory for people engaged in these studies.

Although 21 CFR 820.75(a) refers to the original need for validation and 21 CFR 820.75(b) and (c) refer to ongoing or follow up validations, it is clear that the manufacturer must prepare a single set of documents to allow for revalidations and to allow for revalidations if the process appears to be going out of control or if product quality changes. Each validated process needs to be monitored by checking appropriate parameters to ensure that its validation parameters were being met. If there are multiple validated steps in a process, an appropriate number of tests and test points will need to be checked by in-process testing. It is important to track the exact equipment that was involved in the process validation if it is possible that revalidations might employ equipment that is different from that which was involved in the original validation.

✸ Subpart H—Acceptance Activities ✸

21 CFR 820.80 Receiving, In-Process, and Finished Device Acceptance

21 CFR 820.80(a) General. *Each manufacturer shall establish and maintain procedures for acceptance activities. Acceptance activities include inspections, tests, and other verification activities.*

61. **Material Acceptance Program.** First, a high-level policy document is needed as 21 CFR 820.80 covers the whole of the manufacturer's acceptance program. Basically, this document will say that acceptance activities will be conducted on incoming material, components, in-process material, and finished devices. It should specify who is responsible for the activities and give a summary of the acceptance procedures that are to be performed for each type of material. All incoming, in-process, and finished material must be subject to acceptance procedures, even if the incoming or in-process material is being obtained from a sister division within the same company. In-process material needs to be accepted at certain stages before proceeding with further manufacturing. This document should also require the use of labels, stickers, or tags that will define the acceptance status as given in 21 CFR 820.86. Examples of the labels and their use should be given, and copies should be included in this document as the labels themselves should be controlled documents. The results of these acceptance activities should be documented as given in 21 CFR 820.80(e). Nonconforming material should be handled as defined in either 21 CFR 820.50 or 21 CFR 820.90 as the situation requires. Disposition directions should be written into documents for those sections.

21 CFR 820.80(b) Receiving Acceptance Activities. Each manufacturer shall establish and maintain procedures for acceptance of incoming product. Incoming product shall be inspected, tested, or otherwise verified as conforming to specified requirements. Acceptance or rejection shall be documented.

62. **Incoming Product Acceptance.** This document should describe and specify the contents of a family of documents as follows. For each raw material, product, or component that will be received by the manufacturing site, a document should be prepared that describes the material, names the approved suppliers, and states the requirements for the acceptance of that material into the process flow and release from quarantine. The document should explain how the acceptance requirements were determined and how they address the issue of the safety and efficacy (utility) of the material. It should describe the

method of inspecting or testing the material. If the acceptance testing or inspection is insufficient to completely assess the safety and efficacy of the material, a requirement for a supplier assessment or audit (see 21 CFR 820.22) should be given with a listing of the portions of the supplier's quality systems that should receive particular attention. This document should be the same as or coordinated with the purchasing product specifications required by 21 CFR 820.50(b). Depending on the nature of the material and the testing or inspection that will be required, this document should include a statistically valid sampling plan. Each incoming batch, lot, or unit of raw material or components should be assigned a unique control (lot) number (see 21 CFR 820.60) that will allow the material to be traced through the manufacturing system back to the supplier. The number should be specific, not only to the supplier's lot numbers but to different shipments of the same lot as well. It is almost impossible to ensure that two shipments of material will be exposed to the same environmental and handling conditions. A summary document should be defined. The summary document should contain lot and date specific information on the incoming material as given in 21 CFR 820.80(e) and an acceptance or rejection statement that is signed and dated by the inspector(s) or supervisor of the activity. The summary document would then be placed in the DHR.

A provision should be made for the "urgent use" of incoming material. Urgent use is permissible if the manufacturer has a method for forward tracing of raw material or components of a device. The release of material to production under an urgent use provision should be recorded and noted as a deviation in the manufacturing record. The use of material under an urgent use provision should cause the manufacturing lot to be flagged to prevent the release of finished product before the verification or reviewing acceptance activity has been completed. Release of finished product before the completion of the acceptance activity would be a violation of 21 CFR 820.80(d). Frequent use of material under an urgent use provision is a sign that there are problems in the procurement or production planning function, and auditors should be directed to pay special attention to these areas.

21 CFR 820.80(c) In-Process Acceptance Activities. *Each manu-facturer shall establish and maintain acceptance procedures, where appropriate, to ensure that specified requirements for in-process product are met. Such procedures shall ensure that in-process prod-uct is controlled until the required inspection and tests or other veri-fication activities have been completed, or necessary approvals are received, and are documented.*

63. **In-Process Acceptance Activities.** At certain key points in the manufacturing sequence, in-process acceptance activities should be performed to verify that the manufacturing processes are proceeding correctly and that important parameters are being met before proceeding with the next step. An accep-tance protocol must be written for the in-process product at each of these points. The document should contain the specifi-cations that must be met and, if separate test protocols are not required, references to test procedures or directions on how the tests are to be conducted. For products where the removal or limitation of manufacturing material must be verified (see 21 CFR 820.70(h)), that inspection or testing activity should be included. In addition, the sampling plan and a template for a summary document that will contain lot specific data as re-quired in 21 CFR 820.80(e) should be included. The summary document must be signed and dated by the individual respon-sible for accepting the in-process material. The specifications should conform to any design output requirements for process intermediates. The summary document would then become a part of the DHR.

    In some cases, although sampling takes place during pro-cessing, the testing is such that test results will not be available within a realistic time frame (sterility testing, for example). In these situations, the protocol should state that processing may proceed provided that other criteria are met, but final accep-tance activities should not commence until the lot has passed the in-process test. After all, there is no point to engaging in the expense of final acceptance activities if the lot will fail in-process testing. If the manufacturer has enough experience with the product to be confident that in-process test failure is not likely, then the product may proceed to final acceptance activities, but in no case can the product be granted final acceptance and release until it has cleared all of the in-process test requirements.

It should also be noted that devices that are fairly straightforward or that are produced via rapid, enclosed, continuous processes may not need in-process testing or acceptance activities. This should not be viewed as an invitation to dispense with all in-process testing. Consultation with the FDA should occur before a decision is made to eliminate in-process testing. In some cases, the argument will be advanced that in-process testing can be eliminated because the results are obtained after the process is completed and cannot be used for a "real time" control of the process. This argument misses the point that the idea is to control the totality of the manufacturing of the product, so while the data may, in fact, be too late to affect the processing of one lot, it can be used to prevent future problems with successive lots.

The elimination of in-process testing can lead to costly consequences as some types of testing can be easily performed on a partially assembled device but not on a finished product. Also, in-process testing can often detect upstream problems before expensive parts are installed or labor-intensive actions are performed.

21 CFR 820.80(d) Final Acceptance Activities. *Each manufacturer shall establish and maintain procedures for finished device acceptance to ensure that each production run, lot, or batch of finished devices meets acceptance criteria. Finished devices shall be held in quarantine or otherwise adequately controlled until released. Finished devices shall not be released for distribution until: (1) The activities required in the DMR are completed; (2) the associated data and documentation is reviewed; (3) the release is authorized by the signature of a designated individual(s); and (4) the authorization is dated.*

64. **Final Acceptance Protocol.** The final acceptance protocol for a device should state the specifications that must be met by an acceptable finished device and describe a statistically based sampling plan. The specifications should be based on the design output requirements for the finished device. For most release tests, a simple reference to a testing protocol will suffice, but if the test is simple enough, a description of the procedure could be included in the protocol. In cases where the removal of manufacturing material is important (see 21 CFR 820.70(h)),

the inspection or testing to verify this removal should be specified, unless it was performed as part of an in-process testing program. The acceptance protocol must define the requirements for releasing the product from quarantine. The acceptance criteria and acceptance test requirements should be given in the DMR (see 21 CFR 820.181). In fact the whole purpose of the final acceptance testing should be to show that the manufactured device meets the requirements of the DMR.

Two summary documents should also be described. One will be the usual summary sheet that contains the information required by 21 CFR 820.80(e) for the lot. The equipment used for critical operations and testing of intermediates and the product also needs to be listed and identified in this document. The other document will be a checklist of all of the acceptance documents generated during the course of manufacturing the lot. This document should require a review of all manufacturing activities to verify that all urgent use flags have been removed and all receiving and in-process acceptance activities completed. At the bottom of the document will be a statement saying that the data related to all testing and acceptance activities have been reviewed and found to be satisfactory. Both documents would be signed by the individual having the authority and responsibility to release the lot of finished devices from the manufacturing area. Both of the summary documents should be placed in the DHR.

65. **Quarantine Protocol.** This may be one or more documents depending on the company's procedures and preferences. For the purposes of this section, the document should define how incoming products (raw material, intermediates, and components) are held under quarantine pending acceptance and then released after acceptance. A similar procedure should be given for in-process intermediates with due consideration given to the nature of the process. Hold points and conditions should be defined. With in-process intermediates, special consideration should be given to any needs that are created by the incomplete condition of the product, for instance, a dust sensitive part may still be exposed to the room environment and may need to be covered when the incomplete device is stored. The requirements for holding and release of finished product should also be specified. Stickers, tags or labels that denote the status of quarantined material

should be defined and examples should be shown in this document. This must be done to show the acceptance status as required by 21 CFR 820.86. The document should be fairly specific for the manufacturing site. The location of quarantine areas, as well as the method of quarantine, should be given along with an assignment of the responsibility for releasing the material for the next step in processing. Quarantine release forms should be described for each step. As the movement of product related material is an important activity, the quarantine release forms should be signed and dated by a responsible individual. At this stage, the quarantine sticker or label should be obliterated. This is usually done by placing an acceptance sticker directly over the wording that indicated the material was quarantined. The completed summary forms, containing a summary of the release activities and the results of testing, should become a part of the DHR.

Depending on the company, these are probably not the only quarantine procedures that will be required. Other quarantine documents regarding warehousing procedures, segregation of rejected or returned material, and so on will also be needed, but not by this section of the regulations.

21 CFR 820.80(e) Acceptance Records. *Each manufacturer shall document acceptance activities required by this part. These records shall include: (1) The acceptance activities performed; (2) the dates acceptance activities are performed; (3) the results; (4) the signature of the individual(s) conducting the acceptance activities; and (5) where appropriate the equipment used. These records shall be part of the DHR.*

The requirements of 21 CFR 820.80(e) have been or should have been written into the summary documents described for 21 CFR 820.80(b), (c), and (d) above. A separate document should not be required, if this is done. While not mentioned above, the identification of exactly what was accepted and a comparison between the acceptance criteria and the actual acceptance test results should be given somewhere in the documentation. This comparison usually needs to be summarized with a signed statement to the effect that requirements were met at this step.

21 CFR 820.86 Acceptance Status

Each manufacturer shall identify by suitable means the acceptance status of product, to indicate the conformance or nonconformance of product with acceptance criteria. The identification of acceptance status shall be maintained throughout manufacturing, packaging, labeling, installation, and servicing of the product to ensure that only product which has passed the required acceptance activities is distributed, used, or installed.

Paragraph 21 CFR 820.86 does not appear to require a separate document. Instead, the manufacturer should review the documentation prepared in response to 21 CFR 820.80 for receiving and manufacturing acceptance, 21 CFR 820.90 for nonconforming product, 21 CFR 820.150 for storage, 21 CFR 820.160 for distribution, 21 CFR 820.170 for installation, 21 CFR 820.120 for labeling, and 21 CFR 820.200 for servicing. The object of the review will be to verify the inclusion of instructions to clearly indicate the acceptance status of components and products during the activities mentioned in the paragraph. This could be done with a computer entry or other method that will indicate the acceptance status. Specific labeling is only one of many possible methods. Note that an acceptance can be simply a release for further processing. The whole point here is that product accepted for release must be controlled until it is released to the customer.

This requirement will need a variety of responses. For instance with components, it is common to place a "quarantined" sticker on their packaging upon receipt and then place a "released" sticker directly over the "quarantined" sticker when the component has passed its acceptance testing or review. A similar procedure may be followed for other stages of manufacturing, but it is probably not acceptable when the product reaches its final packaging and labeling stage. At the final stages, it may be necessary to use enclosures such as cages with appropriate tags to denote the status of the enclosed material. Because of the varieties of possible responses to this requirement, it is best to write the procedure directly into the document that controls activities at a given stage, rather than to try to collect all instructions covering all stages into a single document. The manufacturer will find that 21 CFR 820.60 ties into this requirement, as there should be a requirement for identification of the lot, batch, or unit as well as for denoting the acceptance status.

❧ Subpart I— ❧ Nonconforming Product

21 CFR 820.90 Nonconforming Product

21 CFR 820.90(a) Control of Nonconforming Product.   Each manufacturer shall establish and maintain procedures to control product that does not conform to specified requirements. The procedures shall address the identification, documentation, evaluation, segregation, and disposition of nonconforming product. The evaluation of nonconformance shall include a determination of the need for an investigation and notification of the persons or organizations responsible for the nonconformance evaluation and any investigation shall be documented.

   21 CFR 820.3(q) Nonconformity *means the nonfulfillment of a specified requirement.*

66. **Nonconformance Reporting.** The first thing that the document for fulfilling 21 CFR 820.90(a) must do is to require all acceptance testing documents (see 21 CFR 820.80 and 21 CFR 820.86) to refer to this document under "procedures to be followed if the product fails to meet acceptance criteria." Any document that controls an acceptance or release activity should refer to this document. The CGMP definition of product (21 CFR 820.3(r)) should be reviewed before proceeding with this and the following documents.

   The second thing that this document should do is to require that each document that controls an acceptance activity provide instructions for denoting the nonconforming status of the product (see 21 CFR 820.60 and 21 CFR 820.86) at whatever stage the nonconformance was found. It should also require segregation of the nonconforming product from conforming product at that particular stage with specific instructions on the method to be used for the segregation. The segregation should be coordinated with the quarantine activities required for 21 CFR 820.80 and document 65. There should also be a requirement for recording and documenting the ultimate disposition of the nonconforming material.

In the preamble, the FDA provided a useful description of a nonconformity when it stated that "a nonconformity may not always rise to the level of a product defect or failure, but a product defect or failure will always constitute a nonconformity."

The third part of this document should give a general format for a report that will document the nonconformance and provide for an initial evaluation of the cause of the nonconformance. The report should be prepared either by the personnel who discover the nonconformance or by other personnel in the department handling the product when the nonconformance was found. This document will then serve as the basis for an investigation of the nonconformance, and a copy should be provided to the people or organization in which the nonconformance occurred. (Note that the regulation says that the notification should go to the persons or organization responsible for the nonconformance, but that is not always possible before the conclusion of the investigation. The persons or organization really responsible for the nonconformance may actually be several steps upstream from the point where the nonconformance is discovered.)

Once the nonconforming material is segregated and quarantined, the investigation of the nonconformance should then take place as a part of the next activity.

21 CFR 820.90(b) Nonconformity Review and Disposition. **(1)** *Each manufacturer shall establish and maintain procedures that define the responsibility for review and the authority for the disposition of nonconforming product. The procedures shall set forth the review and disposition process. Disposition of nonconforming product shall be documented. Documentation shall include the justification for use of nonconforming product and the signature of the individual(s) authorizing the use.*

67. **Materials Review Board.** In many organizations, nonconforming product is reviewed by a Materials Review Board (MRB). This committee is formed with senior personnel, primarily from

Manufacturing and Quality Assurance. There are usually representatives from Purchasing and Engineering, with participation from other groups as the need arises. This document should create the MRB and assign to the MRB the authority to review nonconformances and dispose of nonconforming product or to accept nonconforming product by concession. The activities of the MRB must be documented. Provisions should be made to review any document that reports a nonconformance and to investigate all related circumstances before any decisions on the disposition of the product are made. In addition to the requirements for justifying any use of nonconforming product, the instructions should require a justification process for any disposition of product, with appropriate dates and signatures for the action. The justifications made should be based upon the results of the investigation of the nonconformance.

Acceptance of material by concession must be documented. In the preamble to the "Working Draft of the CGMP Final Rule," the FDA has stated that the justification for a concession "should be based on scientific evidence and objective decision making, which a manufacturer should be prepared to provide upon request. Such concessions should be closely monitored and not become accepted practice."

21 CFR 820.90(b)(2) *Each manufacturer shall establish and maintain procedures for rework, to include retesting and reevaluation of the nonconforming product after rework, to ensure that the product meets its current approved specifications. Rework and reevaluation activities, including a determination of any adverse effect from the rework upon the product, shall be documented in the DHR.*

21 CFR 820.3(x) Rework *means action taken on a nonconforming product so that it will fulfill the specified DMR requirements before it is released for distribution.*

68. **Control of Rework.** The document for 21 CFR 820.90(b)(2) will irect the preparation of procedures for reworking nonconforming product. Whenever nonconforming product is reworked to correct the nonconformance and produce releasable product, a protocol or procedure needs to be prepared to direct and control the events associated with the reprocessing. For each type of nonconformance, the document should cover the following:

a. The methods and processes to be used in recovering and preparing the product for the reworking and the testing to be done, if any. This should include identification methods for showing that the product is being reworked. These identification methods should be in keeping with 21 CFR 820.90(a) and also 21 CFR 820.60 and 21 CFR 820.86. It will be best if special lot or unit numbers are issued to avoid confusion between material being reprocessed and regular material. The identification of the material as devices that are being reworked needs to be present only during the reworking and may be removed later. The manufacturer may wish to develop a special series of lot numbers that will alert employees to the fact that a product is being reworked, while appearing to be a normal lot number as far as a customer would be concerned. The preparation for reprocessing should follow run sheets that tell what must be done and serve as records of the reprocessing events.

b. The procedures to be followed for the reprocessing should include appropriate identification (21 CFR 820.60) and acceptance status (21 CFR 820.86) notification procedures. The procedures should be in the form of run sheets that will give procedures to be followed as well as serve as a record of events during the reprocessing. Note that one cannot simply write a rework protocol and start reworking. The protocol must be checked against the design requirements (21 CFR 820.30) and also against license statements to see if the reprocessing will violate any provisions or create conflicts with design requirements. Will the reprocessing affect the stability of a component or its reliability? It may be necessary to prepare a license amendment and seek FDA approval before using a particular reprocessing protocol. If nonconformances occur frequently and cannot be controlled through quality assurance procedures, it may be worth the effort to prepare a license amendment for the reprocessing procedure.

c. The reevaluation of the reprocessed product with appropriate in-process testing during the rework and finished product evaluations after reprocessing. This should include any special testing requirements that might arise because of the nature of the nonconformance or of the rework. For instance, if the device is nonconforming due to a sterilization failure, it may mean that additional samples will need to be tested to provide a higher level of confidence after the second sterilization process. The reevaluation should be recorded in the form of a test summary, certificate of analysis, or evaluation sheet that will record the results of tests, refer to the location of the raw data for the tests, and have a final statement of acceptability or rejection of the reprocessed lot. This statement should be signed and dated by personnel who are normally responsible for the release of product for distribution.

d. Any special testing or evaluation procedures that will be needed to see if the reworking had an unusual or unexpected effect on the product. For instance, with a sterilization rework, it may be necessary to check the effect of a second round of heating or irradiation on the stability of certain components. It may not be necessary to do this testing on each reprocessed lot, if validation studies are available showing that the reprocessing does not affect the device in any significant manner. The results of this testing or evaluation should be included in the test summary mentioned previously.

e. A provision that copies of all run sheets and test summaries shall be placed in a device history record pertaining to the particular device and reprocessing operation (see 21 CFR 820.184).

When discussing nonconforming product and its reworking, some individuals like to play semantic games to avoid rules or responsibility. If a document says that a certain procedure constitutes "reworking," some will then justify not using that procedure by stating that they are "reprocessing" the device. In this case, reworking may be defined as starting back at step one and then redoing the whole manufacture of the device, where as reprocessing is where you may only go back to an intermediate step and begin the remanufacture. While it may be fun to play these word games, an encounter with a humorless inspector or auditor can generate grim results. It is best not to play word games and regard any remanufacturing or even additional processing in response to a nonconformance as reworking. Reworking should be distinguished from refurbishing, maintenance, and servicing, but a proliferation of "re-" words probably will not be to the manufacturer's benefit.

※ Subpart J—Corrective ※ and Preventive Action

21 CFR 820.100 Corrective and Preventive Action

21 CFR 820.100(a) Procedures. Each manufacturer shall establish and maintain procedures for implementing corrective and preventive action. The procedures shall include requirements for:

(1) Analyzing processes, work operations, concessions, quality audit reports, quality records, service records, complaints, returned product, and other sources of quality data to identify existing and potential causes of nonconforming product, or other quality problems. Appropriate statistical methodology shall be employed where necessary to detect recurring quality problems;

(2) Investigating the cause of nonconformities relating to product, process, and the quality system;

(3) Identifying action(s) needed to correct and prevent recurrence of nonconforming product and other quality problems;

(4) Verifying or validating the corrective and preventive action to ensure that such action is effective and does not adversely affect the finished device;

(5) Implementing and recording changes in methods and procedures needed to correct and prevent identified quality problems;

(6) Ensuring that information related to quality problems or nonconforming product is disseminated to those directly responsible for assuring the quality of such product or the prevention of such problems; and

(7) Submitting relevant information on identified quality problems, as well as corrective and preventive actions, for management review.

21 CFR 820.100(b) Documented Activities. All activities required under this section, and their results, shall be documented.

69. **Corrective and Preventive Action.** The first document required for corrective and preventive action is one that assigns the activities required in this part to the Quality Assurance/Quality

Control Department (Quality Systems Department?). The responsibility should include gathering the data that will allow the analyses mentioned in 21 CFR 820.100(a)(1) and the investigations in 21 CFR 820.100(a)(2). In contrast to the complaints in 21 CFR 820.198, this part of the regulations applies to process and quality system nonconformities as well as those related to product. Quality system problems such as a lack of training or poor documentation need to be addressed. Potential nonconformities that have been identified through investigations also need to be addressed, as this will be viewed as a preventive action. The activities conducted under 21 CFR 820.100(a) could arise from internal as well as external sources of information. Any trends or systemic problems that are noticed as a result of analyzing service reports (21 CFR 820.200) should be investigated. All devices suspected of possessing nonconformities must be investigated, and the cause of the nonconformities determined when possible, whether or not they have been distributed. Provisions for locating and, if necessary, recalling distributed devices should be made. Failure investigations should be covered also. If a component or the device itself fails to meet requirements, the cause of the failure needs to be investigated before the fact of the failure can be corrected.

If a corrective action can be considered to be a remedial action as defined by 21 CFR 803, there may be a need to report the action to CDRH within a five-day or 30-day period. The manufacturer needs to coordinate actions taken under this section with those required by 21 CFR 803 (the MDR) and 21 CFR 820.198.

The investigations of nonconformities should be performed in concert with the activities under 21 CFR 820.90(b). An analysis of the risk posed by the nonconformity should be performed and recorded. Any problem due to user error will be considered to be a nonconformity as it should have been prevented through risk analysis and human factors engineering during the design of the product. Also, portions of these investigations should be covered by the internal quality audits described in 21 CFR 820.22, and the interaction between the internal quality audits and the activities of this part should be defined. This document should also define the responsibility for notifying all affected parties of the existence of a quality problem. These people would be those responsible for quality and for preventing or otherwise dealing with the problem. The investigation should be recorded and the resulting report should be placed in a file for nonconformances. The statistical methodology to be employed in these reviews should be named here and a detailed description of the procedures should be given under 21 CFR 820.250.

70. **Corrective Action Teams.** Another document needed for 21 CFR 820.100 should assign the responsibility and authority for the formation of corrective action teams (sometimes called CAT teams) to deal with nonconformances and their causes or other quality problems. The CAT should be directed to deal with all quality problems that may be revealed during its investigations, not just the original nonconformity. The object is to prevent and correct poor practices, not just bad product. The CAT team must have the responsibility and authority to effect corrective actions following management review. It is often wise to have sufficient management members on this team so that reviews and approvals can be handled within the team. The document should describe a format that will require a formal memo or other document that names the members of the team, the scope of action, and the goals for the team. The team should be composed of individuals with diverse backgrounds and not be confined just to Quality Assurance or Manufacturing personnel or employees in a single department or classification.

The document should suggest and describe problem-solving techniques that might be used (e.g., Pareto charts, Fishbone diagrams) and also a requirement for a risk assessment of the nonconformity. Statistical methods to be employed should be appropriate for the work at hand. The document should also define the position of the teams within the company's management system and contain a provision for the dissolution of the teams once their goals have been met. The members of the teams should be responsible for communicating relevant information to their respective departments, and for gathering relevant information to the problem from their departments. The CAT will be responsible for the activities needed to comply with the requirements of 21 CFR 820.100(a)(1) to (a)(7). It should consider the possibility of improper or inadequate training, a failure to follow procedures or inadequate procedures, and other possible causes of nonconformance. The CAT should develop methods for assessing the risk and have specific responses for different levels of risk. The CAT must be directed to correct and prevent the recurrence of the nonconformity, and the degree of its actions will depend on the level of risk that is determined to exist. The CAT must be formed and take action even when the nonconformity is the result of the misuse of the device. These points should be covered in this organizing document. The activities of the CAT should be documented and filed with the investigations of the nonconformities.

71. **Corrective Action Requests.** The operational document here will be the corrective action request (CAR). The CAR should be the same document that is used for requesting corrective actions resulting from quality audits (see 21 CFR 820.22). A master document should be created to define the format of a CAR and the actions that will be required to comply with it. A CAR should clearly state the problem that needs correction and contain a requirement for management review upon its issuance. It should request both short- and long-term corrective actions and contain a date for the implementation of at least the short-term corrective action. A CAR can be issued by any person who discovers a situation requiring corrective action. CAT teams usually are formed to act on CARs but may themselves issue CARs.

   CARs are usually two-part documents. The first part was described above. The second part is for a summary of the response to the CAR. It should contain a provision that requires management review of the response and the dissemination of the information to all affected groups within the company. The purpose here is to assure the execution of the corrective action and to ensure management awareness of the problem and its solution. Management should agree that the CAR has been closed to the company's satisfaction. There should be a formal procedure for closing a CAR and for filing the closed document in a file associated with the nonconformance that it addressed.

❋ Subpart K—Labeling ❋ and Packaging Control

21 CFR 820.120 Device Labeling

Each manufacturer shall establish and maintain procedures to control labeling activities.

21 CFR 820.120(a) Label Integrity. *Labels shall be printed and applied so as to remain legible and affixed during the customary conditions of processing, storage, handling, distribution, and, where appropriate, use.*

72. **Label Integrity and Validation.** If labels are purchased from an external source, the purchasing data required under 21 CFR 820.50(b) should clearly specify the label material, ink, printing style, adhesive, and any other information related to the ability of the label to satisfy the requirements of this paragraph. If the labels are prepared by the manufacturer, the same information should be presented to the internal print shop. The information to be presented to the internal print shop should be the result of experimental studies that will be defined by this document. This information and the label contents should have been developed, initially, as a part of the design output (see 21 CFR 820.30 (d) and 21 CFR 820.3(g)). The ability of the label to remain legible and affixed after exposure to common solvents, such as alcohol; to high humidity; to low humidity; to low or high temperatures; and to common cleaning agents or disinfectants should be evaluated along with other, related, factors when deciding upon an acceptable label for the device or its packaging. A useful process is to have an evaluation of label integrity as a part of any stability study or shipping validation or the activities used to meet the requirements of 21 CFR 820.160. Thus, each label should be designed to meet the needs of 21 CFR 820.120(a), and there should be data available to support the selection of a particular label. The writing and style of the label should be aimed at the potential reader. Thus the labeling on a device that is to be

used primarily by elderly individuals may need to be in larger type while a device to be used by children should have a label that uses a simple vocabulary. The document required here should describe the process by which a label will be evaluated, the reports and documentation required, and how the final requirements will be presented. The information developed here, especially the specifications, should be placed in the DHR described in 21 CFR 820.184. The Quality Systems Manual contains a useful table showing the sequence of events in labeling development.

Note that labeling is defined in the Food, Drug and Cosmetics Act in Sections 201(k, l, and m), and the definitions are broad enough that direction inserts, operating and maintenance manuals, reprints of publications, tags, display panels, and advertisements may be considered to be labels. Also, the contents of the labels are covered in Sections 502(f)(1 & 2) of the Act. Other regulations related to labeling will be found in 21 CFR 801, 807, 809, 812, 814, and 1010, depending on the type of device that is being produced. Other requirements will be found in the "Fair Packaging and Labeling Act" and the "Radiation Control for Health and Safety Act." These regulations should be regarded as being incorporated by reference into the quality system regulations when appropriate for a particular device. The manufacturer needs to be aware of the fact that incorrectly prepared labels can lead to the product being classified as being misbranded or possessing false or misleading labeling.

21 CFR 820.120(b) Labeling Inspection.   Labeling shall not be released for storage or use until a designated individual(s) has examined the labeling for accuracy including, where applicable, the correct expiration date, control number, storage instructions, handling instructions, and any additional processing instructions. The release, including the date and signature of the individual(s) performing the examination, shall be documented in the DHR.

73. **Label Copy Verification.** A labeling inspection protocol should be written to cover the requirements of 21 CFR 820.120(b). The protocol should require the activity to take place upon receipt of the labels or just after their printing, depending on the situation for the manufacturer. A sampling procedure should be defined.

The labels should be compared against an approved version of the label copy and the purchase specifications from 21 CFR 820.50(b). Remember that printing on the packaging, packaging inserts, and directions for use may be considered to be labeling. The protocol should specify a summary sheet for each shipment or lot of labels or any other printed material that will accompany the device to the customer. The sheet would include data, such as the label type, number of labels, any control numbers, sampling data, results of the examination, an accounting of the disposition of all labels, and the release with the signature of the responsible individuals. A sample of the label should be attached to the summary sheet. The summary sheet would then become a part of the DHR (21 CFR 820.184). In addition to this section of the CGMPs, there are other requirements for device labels. Devices in general are discussed in 21 CFR 801, and investigational devices are discussed in 21 CFR 812.5. *In Vitro* Diagnostics (IVD) are covered in 21 CFR 809.10(b).

If the labeling is printed directly on the device or packaging, a photograph or other type of verified copy could be attached to the summary sheet, and the inspector will have to conduct an examination at the time and place that the labeling is printed. Also, if optical scanning and recognition are used to verify printing and labeling, an inspector should still periodically perform a visual inspection to confirm the correctness of the labeling and that the scanner is operating properly. The results of these activities would then be entered on the summary sheet.

Automated readers and optical scanners will come into increasing use to verify the proper printing and placement of labels. There is much to be gained in the way of efficiency and speed of operations, but it is important to remember that, like all electronic machines, these devices are subject to errors in programming and false signals that are accepted as real. If labels are verified by using a scanner that is working off the same exemplar that was used for printing the label, it is important to have a human performing a periodic check to make sure that the scanner is not verifying the same incorrect label that the software directed the printer to print. Similarly, periodic checks need to be done to verify the correctness of the instrument's behavior. A microprocessor that "locks up and goes out to lunch" while allowing thousands of units to sail past its reviewing stand must be detected as soon as possible. As with any software-controlled devices used in manufacturing, the software and its performance in the scanner or reader will need to be checked and validated.

21 CFR 820.120(c) Labeling Storage. *Each manufacturer shall store labeling in a manner that provides proper identification and is designed to prevent mixups.*

74. **Label Storage and Issuance.** Basically, labels should be stored and issued in the same manner as is used for any other device component or raw material. This document needs to establish storage conditions for labels with a method for making them readily identifiable while stored. The storage area should be arranged to keep types of labels physically separated and secure, and to generally avoid the possibility of mixups. When the labels are issued for use, there should be a verification activity that will show that the proper number and type of labels were issued from storage and received by the labeling group. Unused labels need to be returned to storage or destroyed through a procedure that verifies the type and number returned or destroyed. The storage environment and security precautions need to be described.

21 CFR 820.120(d) Labeling Operations. *Each manufacturer shall control labeling and packaging operations to prevent labeling mixups. The label and labeling used for each production unit, lot, or batch shall be documented in the DHR.*

A separate document is not needed here, as the manufacturer should place this requirement into the run sheets that control the labeling and packaging operations under 21 CFR 820.70(a). As with any raw material or component a record of the label or labeling and a verification of its suitability for use should be placed in the DHR. Perhaps a document might be written for this activity. An important consideration here is to have manufacturing directions that require a separation of activities, with a "line clear" before and after labeling operations.

Subparagraphs 21 CFR 820.120(c) and (d) appear to be mainly directed at the avoidance of mixups, as improperly labeled devices can produce major problems. However, there is another consideration that should be at least considered when preparing documentation to meet the needs of these subparagraphs. This is the need for monitoring the number of labels used. While devices usually do not have the problems of drugs and biologics in this regard, it is still best if the manufacturer can have some assurance that there is not a large number of uncontrolled labels somewhere in the system. Large numbers of uncontrolled, but legitimate labels, can serve as the basis for fraudulent activities and major mislabeling events. Consequently, the manufacturer will want to monitor the number of labels ordered and the number of labels that are consumed in manufacturing activities.

21 CFR 820.120(e) Control Number. *Where a control number is required by Sec. 820.65, that control number shall be on or shall accompany the device through distribution.*

21 CFR 820.3(d) Control number *means any distinctive symbols, such as a distinctive combination of letters or numbers, or both, from which the complete history of the purchasing, manufacturing, packaging, labeling, and distribution of a unit, lot, or batch of finished devices can be determined.*

Subparagraph 21 CFR 820.120(e) does not require a separate document. If the control number is to be placed on the device itself, this procedure should be a part of the procedures in 21 CFR 820.70 (a). If the number is to be on the label, the specification should be a part of the specifications required by 21 CFR 820.50(b) and 21 CFR 820.120(b). The decision on whether or not to have a control number and its placement should have been covered in the design history under 21 CFR 820.30(c) and (d), and in 21 CFR 820.60 and 21 CFR 820.65. If a control number is used, it is vital to ensure that the entire history of the device, including matters such as the environmental conditions during manufacture, can be determined by using the number.

As a general consideration on the subject of labels, the reader should be aware that labeling issues are responsible for a significant percentage of licensing and product release problems. The wording and design of labels can become an important issue that may impede the progress of a regulatory submission or result in a product recall. As a result, the manufacturer should devote a reasonable amount of time and resources to preparing labels.

21 CFR 820.130 Device Packaging

Each manufacturer shall ensure that device packaging and shipping containers are designed and constructed to protect the device from alteration or damage during the customary conditions of processing, storage, handling, and distribution.

75. **Packaging and Shipping Containers.** The document for complying with 21 CFR 820.130 needs to establish a requirement that the packaging and shipping containers for the device should also undergo design and development generally following the major points given in 21 CFR 820.30 under Design Controls and the design output as given in 21 CFR 820.30(d) and 21 CFR 820.3(g). The idea here is that the packaging and shipping containers need to be designed to meet the requirements of this paragraph and those of 21 CFR 820.60, 21 CFR 820.65, 21 CFR 820.70 (a), 21 CFR 820.70(e), 21 CFR 820.140, and 21 CFR 820.150. If a device is to be sterilized with ethylene oxide, the packaging material must be permeable enough to allow the gas and air to be exchanged. In addition, the manufacturer should remember that printing on packaging and shipping containers may be part of the device labeling and may need to be reviewed for potential regulatory problems. If the packaging is purchased from an external vendor, this vendor should undergo auditing or review like any other supplier. In general, packaging should be regarded as a major device accessory and dealt with in the same manner.

    The packaging should undergo two different types of validation. The first might be looked upon as a process validation. Given the raw material (or components) purchased by the manufacturer, the ability to properly package the device needs to be validated. This activity needs to consider the specifications for the raw material as well as the processing checks that confirm proper packaging. The second validation would be a demonstration that the packaging is capable of satisfying user needs with respect to the device. This will be discussed in more detail.

    If the device is believed to be sensitive to shipping or storage conditions, it would be best to provide for shipping validation studies that will test the ability of the packaging to protect the device during storage, handling, or shipping. Even if the device is considered to be perfectly stable, the manufacturer will want information on some of the fundamental properties of the packaging. Parameters such as burst strength, crush resistance, ability to withstand immersion or moist environments, ability to insulate against temperature extremes, protect against external magnetic fields, or static electricity, and cushioning from physical shock could be considered and, if important, checked by an actual validation study on the packaging. In shipping validations, manufacturers have been known to enclose accelerometers and recording thermometers in their packaging to validate their shipping procedures. Similar studies should be done here.

❋ Subpart L—Handling, Storage, ❋ Distribution, and Installation

21 CFR 820.140 Handling

Each manufacturer shall establish and maintain procedures to ensure that mixups, damage, deterioration, contamination, or other adverse effects to product do not occur during handling.

21 CFR 820.140 does not really require a document of its own. Such a document, if written, would have to be general in nature, while covering all of the handling events that would need to be considered. In some cases, the involvement of the manufacturer could be such that the responsibility for handling may go well beyond the distribution stage. It is better to ensure that the requirements of this paragraph are met by adding them to the documents prepared for complying with 21 CFR 820.70 (a) under Production and Process Controls, 21 CFR 820.150 for Storage, 21 CFR 820.160 for Distribution, 21 CFR 820.170 for Installation, and 21 CFR 820.200 for Servicing.

21 CFR 820.150 Storage

21 CFR 820.150(a) Control of Storage. *Each manufacturer shall establish and maintain procedures for the control of storage areas and stock rooms for product to prevent mixups, damage, deterioration, contamination, or other adverse effects pending use or distribution and to ensure that no obsolete, rejected, or deteriorated product is used or distributed. When the quality of product deteriorates over time, it shall be stored in a manner to facilitate proper stock rotation, and its condition shall be assessed as appropriate.*

21 CFR 820.150(b) Receipt and Dispatch. *Each manufacturer shall establish and maintain procedures that describe the methods for authorizing receipt from and dispatch to storage areas and stock rooms.*

76. **Device Storage and Preservation.** Basically, 21 CFR 820.150 needs to be a document that controls activities in areas where finished or intermediate products will be stored. In addition to the requirements given in 21 CFR 820.150(a) and (b), the handling procedures should conform to the requirements of 21 CFR 820.140. The layout of the storage area needs to be such that "dead pockets," where product can remain while escaping notice (and therefore movement) by stocking personnel, should be eliminated. Products should be clearly identified by name and lot number when in storage. A person standing in the aisle should (with normal vision) be able to read the identification tags of the material in storage. This may mean that special storage tags may need to be employed.

    There must be a strict control over the movement of product into and out of storage areas. This control document should define who has access to storage areas, what procedures must be followed, and what clearances must be obtained before material may be moved into or out of the storage areas. Simply providing a locked room with only one or two keys is not sufficient. If the movement of product into and out of these areas is actually controlled by a different group from the one responsible for physically moving the product, a distribution or production scheduling group for example, a separate document controlling product movement should be written for that group. Unless there are compelling reasons against it, the movement of all product, not just unstable product, through all areas should be based on a first-in first-out (FIFO) method.

    If the product deteriorates over time, a second document should be written to inform the workers of the nature of the instability and the necessity for periodically inspecting or testing the product. Provision should be made for the quarantine of any material that goes past the expected date for an evaluation without receiving an evaluation. This action should be in keeping with the requirements of 21 CFR 820.80(d) and (e), 21 CFR 820.90 and 21 CFR 820.160. The nature of the inspection or testing shall be defined, and a mechanism for reviewing the resulting data and releasing the product for further storage or distribution should be specified, along with the records that will result from this evaluation. The MRB described under 21 CFR 820.90 might be designated as the reviewing group. Data derived from stability studies should be used to define the intervals for checking the product. These intervals should be based on the date of manufacturing and allow for sufficient lead time so that stock can be evaluated, moved, and delivered to the customer before the product can deteriorate to the point where its fitness-for-use will be affected.

21 CFR 820.160 Distribution

21 CFR 820.160(a) Control of Distribution. *Each manufacturer shall establish and maintain procedures for control and distribution of finished devices to ensure that only those devices approved for release are distributed and that purchase orders are reviewed to ensure that ambiguities and errors are resolved before devices are released for distribution. Where a device's fitness-for-use or quality deteriorates over time, the procedures shall ensure that expired devices or devices deteriorated beyond acceptable fitness for use are not distributed.*

77. **Release and Distribution.** The distribution document may be a single document defining a procedure for verifying the approval for release of the device. One part should provide procedures for the review of purchase orders to verify the correctness of distribution orders and to ensure that the requirements given previously are met. Note that these purchase orders are between the manufacturer and its customer in contrast to the purchase orders covered by 21 CFR 820.50 that are between a supplier (vendor) and the manufacturer. A second part may then address the issue of the stability of the

device and the procedures for releasing devices before they deteriorate to the point where they would be unsuitable for use with the patient. Distribution on a first-in first-out (FIFO) basis could be specified with monitoring of the manufacturing dates and last possible distribution dates. Remember that the distributor must allow enough time for receipt and use by the customer before the device's fitness-for-use is severely compromised. The activities under 21 CFR 820.150(b) should be considered if the product deteriorates over time. This document should describe a release form that will summarize the actions taken and the reviews performed prior to the release of the devices. This form should also be the one that contains the data required by 21 CFR 820.160(b).

21 CFR 820.160(b) Distribution Records. *Each manufacturer shall maintain distribution records which include or refer to the location of:*

(1) The name and address of the initial consignee;
(2) The identification and quantity of devices shipped;
(3) The date shipped; and
(4) Any control number(s) used.

78. **Distribution Records.** The document for distribution records should specify and require the entry of the above information in the form referred to for 21 CFR 820.160(a). The distribution group should be given the responsibility to collect, review, and approve the information for inclusion in the distribution records. It should also establish the distribution records as quality records, and specify the documentation group as being responsible for their maintenance and eventual disposal after a specified holding period. The usual rule is to hold records for at least one year past the expiration date of the item. With devices a problem can arise if the manufacturer or some other party engages in a refurbishing activity. In this case, the record-holding period should be extended to cover the refurbished devices, and the distribution records for the refurbished devices should also contain the information required above. This can be especially important if the refurbishing of the device results in using a part or component beyond the length of time originally anticipated during the designing of the device.

If the device is initially delivered to a distribution arm of the manufacturer's corporation, this group should not be considered to be the "initial consignee." It would be best to consider the initial consignee to be the first person outside of the manufacturer's corporation to receive the device. All distribution before this point would represent internal distribution or transfers. If the initial consignee is a distributor or other agent, rather than a user of the device, it might be wise to ask that group to retain records of their consignments of the device in the event that a recall or other tracing becomes necessary. Do not expect distributors or agents to provide the names and addresses of their customers unless absolutely necessary, as they will be afraid of being bypassed for future sales.

The distribution record form used here should be placed in the same file or file set as that which will be used to keep any installation records that are required by 21 CFR 820.170. This will simplify cross-checking and tracing if a quality problem is encountered. There are specific requirements for certain electronic or radioactive devices which are given in 21 CFR 1002.

Note that initial distributors of imported devices bear the same responsibilities as manufacturers. This distributor is expected to maintain complaint files. The initial distributor may also provide maintenance or service for the device, but also has the same responsibilities as a manufacturer of the device.

Even if a control number is not required for purposes of traceability, the manufacturer may want to assign lot or control numbers to aid in inventory and distribution control. These control numbers should be recorded in the DHR. Control numbers can be especially important if the device is unstable or is sensitive to shipping conditions. Control numbers to monitor portions of lots with differing shipping dates or differing shipment routes or carriers can be very useful.

There are certain devices that must be tracked. They include life-sustaining, permanently implanted, or other specifically regulated devices that are subject to the provisions of 21 CFR 821. Section 21 CFR 821.20 lists the devices that must be tracked. For these devices the requirements for traceability go beyond the requirements discussed here, and the reader should review 21 CFR 821 for tracking requirements covering these types of devices.

21 CFR 820.170 Installation

(a) *Each manufacturer of a device requiring installation shall establish and maintain adequate installation and inspection instructions, and where appropriate test procedures. Instructions and procedures shall include directions for ensuring proper installation so that the device will perform as intended after installation. The manufacturer shall distribute the instructions and procedures with the device or otherwise make them available to the person(s) installing the device.*

79. **Installation and Installers.** The first decision to make here is whether or not the device requires installation and, if so, by whom. If the device needs even a simple installation, a set of installation directions should be included with the device. A document needs to be written that specifies the responsibility for preparing the installation directions and how they are to be reviewed. The directions must contain a provision for checking the function of the device after installation to verify proper function, even for a simple installation. Any handling instructions must keep the requirements of 21 CFR 820.140 in mind. The document should contain directions for the review of the installation directions by the company's label copy committee. This is because the installation directions may be considered to be a direction insert and therefore a part of the device labeling.

    If the device is complex enough, a document may need to be written to specify who may install the device, what is necessary to be qualified to install the device, and the procedures for the installation and inspection of the device after installation. This may be prepared in the form of an installation booklet or handbook that will be available to qualified installers. It is important for the manufacturer to be able to show that the device was properly installed at least at the initial installation. The document should specify the training or experience that will be required to qualify a person to be a "qualified installer." A mechanism for identifying and tracking qualified installers will also be needed. If the company itself provides the training and certification for the qualified installers, this will help considerably in tracking the installers and obtaining their cooperation for recordkeeping and future developments regarding the devices.

(b) *The person installing the device shall ensure that the installation, inspection, and any required testing are performed in accordance with the manufacturer's instructions and procedures and shall document the inspection and any test results to demonstrate proper installation.*

80. **Installation Instructions.** It is clear that the manufacturer needs to distribute the installation instructions with the device so that a third party installer may also install the device properly. In these situations, the manufacturer may not have access to or receive copies of installation reports, even when their preparation and return to the manufacturer are specified in the installation directions. In these situations the FDA will not expect the manufacturer to have copies of the installation records, but FDA will expect such information to be available from the third party installers (since they have now become manufacturers) once they have been identified. The requirements of 21 CFR 820.170(b) will apply to these organizations. Installers may be considered to be people who process a finished device, and therefore fall under the definition of a *manufacturer* (see 21 CFR 820.3(o)). This means that they are subject to FDA inspection, and their records can also be reviewed.

This document should contain the inspection checklist or verification procedure that will verify the proper functioning of the device after installation. For a simple device with a simple installation, it may not be necessary to have a separate document, and these directions could be included with the installation directions. For more complex devices, a formal installation qualification (IQ) procedure may be required, with inspection verifications limited to devices of lesser complexity or criticality. In any case, a record that contains the information verifying proper installation by a qualified installer must be described and its return to the manufacturer specified. This could be something as simple as a postcard with a check off and signature. The manufacturer should maintain these records with the distribution documents of 21 CFR 820.160. The document that describes this verification document should also require a periodic review to see if there are patterns of installation difficulties. These records should be available for complaint review to see if there are problems related to particular installers. In addition, the records of the installation inspection must be available for FDA review.

❋ Subpart M—Records ❋

21 CFR 820.180 General Requirements

All records required by this part shall be maintained at the manufacturing establishment or other location that is reasonably accessible to responsible officials of the manufacturer and to employees of FDA designated to perform inspections. Such records, including those not stored at the inspected establishment, shall be made readily available for review and copying by FDA employee(s). Such records shall be legible and shall be stored to minimize deterioration and to prevent loss. Those records stored in automated data processing systems shall be backed up.

21 CFR 820.180(a) Confidentiality. *Records deemed confidential by the manufacturer may be marked to aid FDA in determining whether information may be disclosed under the public information regulation in part 20 of this chapter.*

21 CFR 820.180(b) Record Retention Period. *All records required by this part shall be retained for a period of time equivalent to the design and expected life of the device, but in no case less than 2 years from the date of release for commercial distribution by the manufacturer.*

21 CFR 820.180(c) Exceptions. *This section does not apply to the reports required by Sec. 820.20(c) Management review, Sec. 820.22 Quality audits, and supplier audit reports used to meet the requirements of Sec. 820.50(a) Evaluations of suppliers, contractors, and consultants, but does apply to procedures established under these provisions. Upon request of a designated employee* *of FDA, an employee in management with executive responsibility shall certify in writing that the management reviews and quality audits required under this part, and supplier audits where applicable, have been performed and documented, the dates on which they were performed, and that any required corrective action has been undertaken.*

Although there are several documents needed here, 21 CFR 820.180 is being taken all at once, as its parts are interrelated, and each paragraph will affect any document prepared as a part of these requirements.

81. **Records Group.** The first document for 21 CFR 820.180 needs to establish a records maintenance function. Normally, this group will be the same as or a part of the documentation control department. This is useful, as the distinction between a regular document and a record is not always clear and the documents and records need to be maintained in the same way. If one looks at the definition given for *record* it is clear that any document, data, or report generated in meeting the requirements of 21 CFR 820 will fall under the definition of "records required by this part" and need to be stored, handled, and maintained as described in this paragraph. The document control group should be assigned the responsibility for classifying records, assigning record numbers, and storing the records, including documents maintained for purposes of continuity or history. Basically, this needs to be the same group that is created to meet the requirements of 21 CFR 820.40 and described in Part I, but now, the responsibility for records is added. If possible, this document should be combined with the one generated in response to 21 CFR 820.40.

    The records group should not be responsible for checking on the validity of the information presented to it, but it should be responsible for checking documents to control the proper usage of templates and standard formats and for insisting that documents be properly executed, with all blanks filled in and all questions answered. They should also be responsible for reviewing submitted documents against basic standards for written English, and insisting that the documents and records meet basic requirements for clarity in syntax, spelling, and grammar. Many manufacturers have a documentation system that is almost useless, because procedures and records are so poorly written that they are virtually incomprehensible. When the employee who created the poorly written record leaves the company, the document really becomes incomprehensible. In these cases, the onus should be on the supervisory employees who accepted the document. It is reasonable to expect employees to be able to write at least at the high school level, and it can save considerable amounts of time and money to have clearly written documents available for auditors, inspectors, and future employees.

82. **Records Storage.** The records group needs to have a storage area that is secure and have procedures to keep the records secure and to prevent deterioration. Automated data processing system records are usually backed up by having hard copies stored with handwritten or printed documents. If possible, especially if the whole documentation system is software driven, there should be a mechanism for periodically backing up the whole system and storing the electronic backup in a remote location off the immediate grounds of the manufacturing plant. In a software driven system, the main program itself should be backed up and stored. This is due to the fact that, even with common systems, there will be some customizing of the program to meet the local needs of the manufacturer's procedures and network. In the event of a disaster, the recovery could be lengthened if an unmodified program has to be loaded and re-customized before the backup copies of documents and records could be loaded. Again, as with all software driven systems, this documentation system will need to be validated.

The storage area should be fireproof with an automatic fire extinguisher system. It should be temperature and humidity controlled with provisions made for monitoring or recording of temperature and humidity readings at daily intervals. In this, the document storage area should be no different from any other storage area that the manufacturer has. In fact this storage area should be able to satisfy the requirements of 21 CFR 820.150 if one substitutes the word document for product. The foregoing is, of course, the ideal system. Most real situations fall short of this, because company management often does not appreciate the importance of the documentation system and will not invest the funds needed for a good system. Because of this, it is usually wise to have a backup storage site at a location remote from the location of the primary set of documents.

In the event of a disaster, the manufacturer's documents will play a key role in its ability to recover rapidly and resume production. The most common disaster is fire, but earthquakes, tornadoes, hurricanes, floods, and explosions are also possibilities, depending on the manufacturer's circumstances. The role of the documentation system should be recognized in the manufacturer's disaster recovery plan. The documents will provide the information needed for rebuilding and designing facilities, replacing ruined equipment, securing new raw material and components, and training replacement personnel. Remote storage should be located at a place that one would not expect to be involved in the same disaster that might affect the primary location. If it is within the same zone for a particular type of disaster, then one site should be "hardened" to withstand the expected disaster. At the same time, the remote site should be accessible so that updates and new documents can be routinely deposited there.

Large corporations often have divisions located in different geographic regions serve as remote locations for each other, with electronic document file transfers over a company network. Small companies often use the garage or extra bedroom of a management employee who lives farthest from the plant. This can create problems from a security standpoint, especially if the particular employee becomes disgruntled. It is preferable to rent a storage locker or room, if the company can afford it. Storage in the form of microfilm or electronic media is usually best to minimize the space needed at the remote location.

83. **FDA Review and Confidentiality.** A prime consideration is in making the records available for review and copying by FDA employees. The FDA will interpret copying to mean photocopying or printing of computer files. A policy needs to be written to cover the needs generated by these regulations. First, the

need for "readily available" documents needs to be addressed. The documents need to be available on site as hard copies. Documents stored at remote locations could be made available via modem, e-mail, or by transmission over a company-wide network. These are the procedures usually employed for active or current documents. Inactive, obsolete, or archived documents may take longer to retrieve, and the usual standard for these is that they must be available within 24 hours of the request. The FDA expects the documents to be available during the course of an inspection, and even with a foreign manufacturer who has records at a remote location, the records need to be produced by the next working day. If there are problems due to the effects of time zones, a second day might be allowed, but it is not wise to rely upon this.

Second, confidentiality needs to be addressed. Documents copied or reviewed by the FDA can become available to the public under Freedom of Information or other public access procedures. However, certain types of documents are considered confidential, and the FDA is supposed to respect that confidentiality, if the manufacturer notifies them of that fact. The "part 20 of this chapter" that is referred to in 21 CFR 820.180(a) is 21 CFR 20 (Public Information). This part should be reviewed when preparing this policy. There should be explicit directions requiring a review by a designated senior manager before a document is furnished to an FDA employee. A method such as a rubber stamp with large red block letters for marking documents to indicate confidentiality should be specified. The manufacturer should have well-defined policies on what are and are not confidential documents or information. Documents in files should already be marked and electronic documents should carry the "confidential" designation as part of the document file. The middle of an inspection is no time to be deciding on the confidentiality of a document. Also, routinely designating all documents as being confidential tends to dilute its seriousness and can lead to employees disregarding the designation.

There are also certain special documents that are protected from review by FDA employees. These are the management reviews in 21 CFR 820.20(c), the internal quality audits in 21 CFR

820.22, and the supplier evaluation documents (external audits and others) prepared for 21 CFR 820.50(a). These are protected, because it was felt that respondents or auditees would be less candid and cooperative if they thought that the information they provided would find its way to the FDA. This does not give the manufacturer a license to disregard the regulations. The FDA may still require a company executive to certify in writing that the reviews, audits, and evaluations did take place on certain dates and that corrective actions were taken. The FDA may also review the procedural documents for these processes and determine their adequacy.

Certain other documents, such as personnel documents, are also considered confidential. While not mentioned here in the CGMPs, these documents are covered by other regulations, and their status must be carefully preserved. For instance, FDA inspectors or other auditors may ask to see training records for certain individuals; in this case, it is very important to present only the training records and not entire personnel files. The training record should be available for review, but the personnel file contains confidential information and public disclosure could have severe consequences for the employer. For this reason, the policy document must clearly specify those documents that are confidential, and the documentation system must clearly differentiate these documents so that inadvertent disclosure cannot occur. The confidential portion of the personnel records, for instance, should be maintained by the Human Resources (Personnel) group while the training records are placed into the CGMP record files.

84. **Record Retention.** A record retention policy needs to be written to define record retention times for all of the documents required under 21 CFR 820. The record retention period defined in 21 CFR 820.180(b) should be regarded as a minimum time. Also, different classes of documents will need to be retained for different times. Documents such as those in the device history record (DHR) are specific to a product lot and may expire with the lot, but the documents in the device master record (DMR) or the design history file (DHF) may be needed as long as the particular design is being manufactured. Also, as the

manufacturing process evolves, documents in the DMR may need to be removed and replaced, while the contents of the DHF may not change. Documents that are made obsolete by changes in the manufacturing process may need to be maintained as long as an active DHR exists that refers to the use of that document or record. Every document should be periodically reviewed (possibly a two-year cycle) to see if it reflects current practice or is really needed to support manufacturing. Obsolete documents should be archived and then purged from the system that contains active documents.

Although the regulation only requires the retention of records for a time equivalent to the design and expected life of the device or no less than two years, the manufacturer may wish to keep the records for periods beyond the minimum period. This can be useful if independent refurbishers are known to be prolonging the use of a device or if outdated devices are continuing to be used. Also, if there are questions of long-term health effects due to the action of the device or one of its components, it may be beneficial to the manufacturer to have data available on the original manufacturing of the device. Some procedural documents should be retained for historical purposes, especially if there has been an evolution in the design or the manufacturing process. The space requirements for long-term record storage could be addressed through microfilming, scanning, or translation into electronic media.

21 CFR 820.181 Device Master Record

Each manufacturer shall maintain device master records (DMR's). Each manufacturer shall ensure that each DMR is prepared and approved in accordance with Sec. 820.40. The DMR for each type of device shall include, or refer to the location of, the following information:

21 CFR 820.3(j) Device master record (DMR) *means a compilation of records containing all the procedures and specifications related to a specific finished device, as required by this part.*

21 CFR 820.3(g) Design output: The final portion of this definition states, *"The finished design output will be the basis for the* **device master record."**

Therefore, the FDA considers the information listed in 21 CFR 820.181(a), (b), (c), and (d) to be parts of the design output of 21 CFR 820.30(d).

Basically the DMR will contain the documents that tell how the device is to be manufactured, while the DHR will tell what was done to manufacture a specific lot of the device. While 21 CFR 820.181 allows the use of a simple reference to the location of documents, it is probably best for the DMR to be a document location with actual copies of documents that are designated as being in the DMR. The use of hard copies is better when actively working with the documents. If the manufacturer has an electronic documentation system, however, the following documents should contain document codes or designators that will identify a specific document as being a part of the DMR. The DMR is really a file that contains the instructions and specifications on how to manufacture and distribute a device. It contains all of the procedures related to the device and the current manufacturing specifications that represent the transfer of the design specifications to production. All material and process specifications, including raw material and component specifications, should be a part of the DMR along with all procedures related to manufacturing, QA/QC, packaging, labeling, installation, maintenance, and servicing the device.

Useful guidance concerning the DMR can be found in the Preamble to the "Working Draft of the CGMP final Rule" and also in the Quality Systems Manual. The final design output that is contained within the DHF serves as the basis for the DMR. All of the design outputs should be represented in the DMR. The final design output includes the final device and process specifications and drawings, and all instructions and procedures used for purchasing, production, installation, maintenance, and servicing.

The regulation also requires a "qualified individual(s)" to prepare the DMR. This would suggest that a Product Development Team or a Product Management Team would receive the assignment. The team and its leader would need to approve the final DMR and sign off on its acceptance. In addition, this group or individual should be responsible for controlling any changes to the DMR. Changes to the DMR should be reviewed and approved through the company's change control procedures.

21 CFR 820.181(a) Device Specifications. *Device specifications including appropriate drawings, composition, formulation, component specifications, and software specifications;*

85. **Device Specifications.** A document defining device specifications should be prepared. List the specifications with appropriate references to the location of the documents that set the specifications. The references would be documents such as formulation study reports, design output documents, software validation studies, failure analysis studies, and other reports and studies that support the specifications present in this part of the DMR. The DMR should contain the latest versions of these specifications while older versions, including older software code, are held in the DHF. Since the contents of the DMR should be comprehensible to the workers employed in manufacturing the device, any special documents such as circuit diagrams or engineering drawings may create needs for special training to ensure the ability of the workers to understand the documents.

21 CFR 820.181(b) Process Specifications. *Production process specifications including the appropriate equipment specifications, production methods, production procedures, and production environment specifications;*

86. **Production Process Specifications.** This document should list documents related to the manufacturing process and the equipment specifications for each item, and the production environment specifications with references to the documents that support those specifications, including process validations, equipment qualifications, and cleaning validations. Processing documents such as production run sheets, and production environment monitoring records should be included along with any in-process testing specifications.

21 CFR 820.181(c) Quality Assurance. *Quality assurance procedures and specifications including acceptance criteria and the quality assurance equipment to be used;*

87. **QA Procedures and Specifications.** This document should list the quality assurance/quality control test, sampling, and monitoring procedures, the intermediate and finished product re-

lease specifications, and a description of the apparatus used, especially gauges or other devices that are specific to the device that is being manufactured. These listed procedures should be those specific to the device and do not need to include general quality assurance procedures such as audit protocols or procedures for contract review.

21 CFR 820.181(d) Packaging and Labeling. *Packaging and labeling specifications, including methods and processes used; and*

88. **Packaging and Labeling Specifications and Studies.** This document should refer to the location of packaging design studies (see 21 CFR 820.130) that support the final packaging and packaging specifications to be used. The specifications themselves should be a part of the DMR. The labeling specifications should describe the wording, method of labeling, type of label, and methods by which the labels are to be prepared. Methods of printing or label processing procedures should be specified. Also, the quality assurance acceptance procedures and specifications for labels and prototypes should be described. This activity should be coordinated with that in 21 CFR 820.120. All documents generated for compliance with 21 CFR 820.120 or 21 CFR 820.130 should be considered for placement in the DMR,

21 CFR 820.181(e) Installation, Maintenance, and Servicing Procedures and Methods.

89. **Installation, Maintenance, and Servicing.** This document could be a simple listing and collection of other documents. Most of these could be represented by copies of documents supplied to customers, installers, and field service representatives. The information needed here should be obtained from the documents prepared to meet the needs of 21 CFR 820.170 and 21 CFR 820.200. The documents themselves could be placed in the DMR.

21 CFR 820.184 Device History Record

Each manufacturer shall maintain device history records (DHR's). Each manufacturer shall establish and maintain procedures to ensure that DHR's for each batch, lot, or unit are maintained to demonstrate that the device is manufactured in accordance with the DMR and the requirements of this part. The DHR shall include, or refer to the location of, the following information:

(a) *The dates of manufacture;*
(b) *The quantity manufactured;*
(c) *The quantity released for distribution;*
(d) *The acceptance records which demonstrate the device is manufactured in accordance with the DMR;*
(e) *The primary identification label and labeling used for each production unit; and*
(f) *Any device identification(s) and control number(s) used.*

21 CFR 820.3(i) Device history record *means a compilation of records containing the complete production history of a finished device.*

90. **Device History Record (DHR).** This is basically a lot-specific file or the production lot record. The DHRs will form a class of documents with each DHR being based on the requirements of a DMR. A document is needed to establish the contents of the DHR. This document could start by specifying a summary sheet that contains the information requested in (a)–(f) above with explanations of differences between (b) and (c) and affixed copies of (e). This summary sheet could include the results of lot release testing and inspections and should also identify the DMR that it is based upon.

The DHR should then include lot-specific documents or information required by the particular DMR. These would be the production run sheets, environmental monitoring records for the lot, and copies of quality assurance test reports. The testing and acceptance results for components and sterilization steps should also be included. Other documents that are not specifically required, but would be useful in the DHR, would be any deviation notices or discrepancy statements that were in effect during the manufacture of the lot and the results of any test failure investigations. A document summarizing the final review of production records and test results prior to the release of a lot should be included in the DHR.

In addition, other sections of these regulations specify documents or information to be included in the DHR. These are as follows:

A. The *acceptance records* and specifications given in 21 CFR 820.50 and 820.80(e).

B. The *reprocessing and reevaluation* records specified in 21 CFR 820.90(b)(2).

C. The *labeling inspection* release document specified in 21 CFR 820.120(b).

21 CFR 820.186 Quality System Records

Each manufacturer shall maintain a quality system record (QSR). The QSR shall include, or refer to the location of, procedures and the documentation of activities required by this part that are not specific to a particular type of device(s), including, but not limited to the records required by Sec. 820.20. Each manufacturer shall ensure that the QSR is prepared and approved in accordance with Sec. 820.40.

21 CFR 820.3(v) Quality system *means the organizational structure, responsibilities, procedures, processes, and resources for implementing quality management.*

91. **Quality System Documents.** Most of the requirements of 21 CFR 820.186 are already covered by the procedures and documents for all of the activities covered by 21 CFR 820. The idea here seems to be to separate the quality documents from device specific or manufacturing documents. More specifically, the documents generated for 21 CFR 820.20 as well as 21 CFR 820.5 should be considered for inclusion in this system of documents. The documents should be grouped into major subdivisions where possible. These would be groups such as the Device History Record, Internal Quality Audits, and Equipment Maintenance Records. The specific documents to be included in the QSR should be general documents that relate to a company's quality system without specific reference to a type or lot of devices. For instance, a document on how to conduct a CGMP-based quality audit would be acceptable, but an audit document describing a manufacturing audit on the assembly of a device should be placed elsewhere.

21 CFR 820.198 Complaint Files

21 CFR 820.198(a) Maintain Files. Each manufacturer shall maintain complaint files. Each manufacturer shall establish and maintain procedures for receiving, reviewing, and evaluating complaints by a formally designated unit. Such procedures shall ensure that:

(1) All complaints are processed in a uniform and timely manner;

(2) Oral complaints are documented upon receipt; and

(3) Complaints are evaluated to determine whether the complaint represents an event which is required to be reported to FDA under part 803 or 804 of this chapter, Medical Device Reporting.

21 CFR 820.198(b) Review and Evaluate Files. Each manufacturer shall review and evaluate all complaints to determine whether an investigation is necessary. When no investigation is made, the manufacturer shall maintain a record that includes the reason no investigation was made and the name of the individual responsible for the decision not to investigate.

21 CFR 820.198(c) Review and Investigate. Any complaint involving the possible failure of a device, labeling, or packaging to meet any of its specifications shall be reviewed, evaluated, and investigated, unless such investigation has already been performed for a similar complaint and another investigation is not necessary.

21 CFR 820.198(d) MDR Complaints. Any complaint that represents an event which must be reported to FDA under part 803 or 804 of this chapter shall be promptly reviewed, evaluated, and investigated by a designated individual(s) and shall be maintained in a separate portion of the complaint files or clearly identified. In addition to the information by Sec. 820.198(e), records of investigation under this paragraph shall include a determination of:

(1) Whether the device failed to meet specifications;

(2) Whether the device was being used for treatment or diagnosis; and

(3) The relationship, if any, of the device to the reported incident or adverse event.

21 CFR 820.198(e) Record of Investigations. When an investigation is made under this section, a record of the investigation shall be maintained by the formally designated unit identified in paragraph (a) of this section. The record of investigation shall include:

(1) The name of the device;
(2) The date the complaint was received;
(3) Any device identification(s) and control number(s) used;
(4) The name, address, and phone number of the complainant;
(5) The nature and details of the complaint;
(6) The dates and results of the investigation;
(7) Any corrective action taken; and
(8) Any reply to the complainant.

21 CFR 820.198(f) Location of Complaint Unit. When the manufacturer's formally designated complaint unit is located at a site separate from the manufacturing establishment, the investigated complaint(s) and the record(s) of investigation shall be reasonably accessible to the manufacturing establishment.

21 CFR 820.198(g) Non-U.S. Complaint Unit. If a manufacturer's formally designated complaint unit is located outside of the United States, records required by this section shall be reasonably accessible in the United States at either:

(1) A location in the United States where the manufacturer's records are regularly kept; or
(2) The location of the initial distributor.

21 CFR 820.3(b) Complaint means any written, electronic, or oral communication that alleges deficiencies related to the identity, quality, durability, reliability, safety, effectiveness, or performance of a device after it is released for distribution.

The complaint files section is long and complex. It will require several interlocking documents, and these documents must be carefully crafted and reviewed. The reason for this is that documents related to complaints will be subject to review by regulatory agencies and customer representatives. In the case of product liability actions, the documents may undergo legal review and may become items of evidence.

A complaint may arise from just about any source and be transmitted via just about any communication mechanism. The manufacturer must be sensitive to all complaints and be sure that all potential complaints can be captured and reviewed.

92. **Complaint Policy.** The first document on complaint files should be a company policy document that basically states that all complaints, including oral complaints, shall be immediately reviewed, evaluated, and investigated. It should be noted that a complaint can arise from just about any source, but it must satisfy the definition of 21 CFR 820.3(b) to be considered to be a complaint. The first action required here will be to determine if an actual complaint has been made. The responsibilities for these actions must be clearly stated. The implications of 21 CFR 820.198(b), (c), and (d) are such that this policy must be established and followed by any prudent manufacturer. Although 21 CFR 820.198(b) suggests that an investigation may not be necessary, it is difficult to see how the manufacturer will determine this without some sort of minimal investigation to begin with. In turn 21 CFR 820.198(c) requires the review, evaluation, and investigation of any sensible complaint, and 21 CFR 820.198(d) and 21 CFR 803 dictate immediate action under certain circumstances. This then places a requirement on the manufacturer to conduct an immediate review and evaluation to see if critical circumstances are present. Even a conclusion that a complaint has not been made, should be recorded and justified. If the communication sounded important enough to be considered then it should be considered to have been important enough to record. Remember that, should matters degenerate into a product liability action, the manufacturer is more likely to be damned for what may appear to be an inadequate response than for an overreaction.

93. **Complaint Unit.** Depending on the size of the unit or the complexity of the manufacturer's product lines more than one document covering complaint units may be required here. For the small manufacturer with a highly reliable product, the complaint unit may be a single person within the quality assurance function. In fact the complaint unit may be simply an assignment of responsibilities to an existing position or unit. A large manufacturer with many product lines, producing a large

number of devices per year, may require a fully independent unit or a separate unit for each device. Because of the quality assurance aspects of complaints, this unit should be a part of the quality systems department, particularly in the documentation group, but companies have been known to place the unit under Sales, Marketing, Customer Service, or Clinical Affairs.

When considering the physical location of the unit, the manufacturer must remember to consider the provisions of 21 CFR 820.198(f) and (g). In particular, foreign manufacturers need to designate an agent in the U.S. who will be responsible for reporting to the FDA under the MDR provisions of 21 CFR 803 or 21 CFR 804, if the device is subject to these requirements. This agent should also be responsible for the reports required under this section of the CGMP.

If at all possible, the complaint unit should be the central point for receiving complaints and for responding to regulatory agencies and the complainant. If a complaint results in a request for a corrective action (CAR), the CAR and its subsequent closure should be monitored by the complaint unit. Corrective Action Teams (CAT) formed in response to CARs should have representatives from the complaint unit on them. The CARs and reports from CATs should be on file in the complaint unit as well as with the company records. It is certainly not wise to have multiple units fielding and responding to complaints as the chance for matters falling into cracks or for generating conflicting or inappropriate responses increases geometrically. This unit does not need to be the group that conducts the reviews and evaluations. The complaint handling unit should coordinate the review and evaluation of the complaint by clinical, technical, manufacturing, and quality assurance functions, with clear responsibilities and time requirements set forth.

The complaint unit should also receive copies of servicing and maintenance reports in a timely manner. There are times when a customer's request for service is really a complaint over a malfunction. The complaint handling unit needs to review all service reports to see if they really represent complaints about malfunctions. At the very least, the complaint handling unit should review and monitor the service reports to see if there are any unexpected patterns that develop in regard to service requests. Any service report that indicates that service was requested because of a death, injury, or potential hazard to safety must be regarded as a complaint and processed as such.

The timing of this unit's work needs to be defined. Subparagraph 21 CFR 820.198(d) specifies an immediate review, evaluation, and investigation by designated individuals, and 21 CFR 803 and 21 CFR 804, which cover similar types of events, require a report to FDA within five days of the receipt of a complaint related to a death, serious injury, or hazard to safety. The Quality Systems Manual contains an extended discussion on the requirements of the MDR (21 CFR 803) that should be integrated into the requirements of 21 CFR 820.198. There is a need for MDR Event Files (MEFs) that contain the information acquired or referenced and the actions taken while the MDR was investigated. The MEF needs to be maintained for two years from the date of the event or for the expected life of the device whichever is longer. Consequently, MEFs may be regarded as a subset of the complaint files.

The document should also describe provisions for a quick preliminary review of the complaint to see if it falls under the requirements of 21 CFR 820.198(d) or 21 CFR 803 and 21 CFR 804 which are the Medical Device Reporting (MDR) regulations. Every device manufacturer should review 21 CFR 803 as it contains specific reporting provisions for certain devices that will require the creation of other documents beyond those described here. The MDR regulations (21 CFR 803) contain additional provisions and are somewhat different from 21 CFR 820.198(d). The MDR (21 CFR 803) covers the reporting of device failures or malfunctions that lead to death or serious injury or could cause death or serious injury if the event were to recur. The company must report the event to the FDA by telephone within five days of the receipt of the complaint, with a written report to follow within fifteen days. Thus, the procedures for complaint receiving and reviewing must contain provisions for a rapid review by a medically qualified individual (preferably someone with knowledge derived from the clinical trials of the device) and also by a technologist or engineer (preferably someone familiar with the failure mode evaluations that were done during the development of the device). The document should establish a mechanism for passing the information to these reviewers or their backups (each reviewer needs a backup who will not go on vacation or go on a business trip or, hopefully, even get sick, at the same time as the primary reviewer). There should then be a mechanism to insure an immediate review and a response within five working days of the date the complaint was received. At the time this book was being prepared, there were indications that the five-day rule would be relaxed. The reader should check the current requirements under 21 CFR 803.53.

The reason for the two-fold evaluation is the potential for future consequences. Given that the device is a medical device, one may expect that the patients who use or are exposed to the device will be in certain defined medical conditions. It is important to know, medically, if the patient's condition after the device failure or malfunction, combined with the patient's state before the event could lead to serious consequences and, eventually, serious injury. The problem here is that the initial complaint report may describe what appear to be mild consequences for the patient. A medically qualified individual is needed to determine if these apparently mild consequences may be a forerunner of serious consequences. Similarly, an apparently inconsequential failure or malfunction may be an indicator of a developing potential for a catastrophic failure of the device, or the failure may have fortuitously resulted in mild consequences and, in the process, revealed a potential for seriously injuring the patient. An individual who is familiar with the technical functioning of the device will be needed for this evaluation.

Because of the need for a special response to failures and malfunctions that may have serious medical consequences, the mechanisms for reviewing and evaluating complaints should be set up to first determine if a complaint is medical in nature. Remember that the determination that a complaint is not medical in nature is, in itself, a medical decision. Consequently, a medically qualified individual should perform the first, preliminary review. A technically qualified individual who is familiar with the function of the device should always conduct a second review of all complaints, since even the medical complaints must be understood within the context of the functioning of the device.

94. **Complaint Analysis.** If the complaint handling unit is a part of the quality systems function, it should produce periodic summaries of the complaints with trend analyses for different classes. If the complaint unit is a part of another group, such as Marketing or Customer Service, the information needed for the summaries and trending should be provided to the Quality Assurance group responsible for monitoring quality related manufacturing parameters. A document establishing this responsibility and specifying the information to be gathered and reported should be written. Data related to servicing under 21 CFR 820.200 should also be reported to this group. The document should also specify any statistical procedures (to be defined under 21 CFR 820.250) that will be followed. The distribution of the summary should also be specified to ensure review by appropriate management personnel.

95. **Complaint Reports.** The manufacturer should then define the documents to be held in the complaint files. These complaint reports could be preprinted forms or at least a preset format that would talk the preparer through a series of questions that will best describe the complaint and gather the information that the manufacturer will need to respond to the complaint. The information required by 21 CFR 820.198(e)(1)–(5) must be requested. In these days of computerized forms, a template that could be called up on a computer screen would be useful, especially if the answers to the questions were, in turn, automatically entered into a database that could be used for monitoring, tracking, and trending of complaints. A receptionist or other person could use such a form to document oral complaints such as those that might be received through a special complaint telephone number. Since oral complaints are often received by field personnel, such as sales representatives or repair personnel, a training program should be specified for these individuals, and copies of the blank complaint report form should be provided to them. These

activities would be specified under a section of this document covering the mechanisms for receiving complaints.

Because the complaints can provide an inspector or auditor with a quick route into the deficiencies of a manufacturer's quality system, the manufacturer should not be surprised if a review of these complaint files is routinely requested by these individuals. The wise manufacturer will be sure to include in the file a statement on how the complaint was handled and any actions that resulted from the complaint. The idea here is to be sure that the company did respond to every complaint, even ones that were considered to be trivial.

In keeping with 21 CFR 820.198(d) a designator or physical separation should be set up to segregate routine complaint files from those that are related to a death, injury, or safety hazard. Because of the serious consequences arising from misclassification or misfiling, a redundant system should be used. For instance, the report might be coded by applying a colored tape and then physically placed in a particular type of colored file folder. For computer use, the document might be given a special designator or file number, and a special key word could be inserted into its name.

In addition to the information required by 21 CFR 820.198(e)(1)–(5), the form should contain certain additional information such as the following:

❖ A prominent statement with a check-off box or other prominent designator that will indicate whether or not the complaint pertains to a death, injury, of hazard to safety.
❖ The time the complaint was received.
❖ The name and signature of the employee who received the complaint.
❖ The serial number or other identifier for the complaint. The idea here is that each complaint should have a unique identification. This could be a simple sequential number, or it could be a number coded by date or device type. The manufacturer's preferences and past practices should be the guide.
❖ The route by which the complaint was received. If possible, all parties involved in the transmission of the complaint should be identified and the sequence of events noted. Although most of the complaints will be received through

the manufacturer's complaint line, there will be complaints received through unusual channels, such as the service department or sales representatives. It is important to determine if these are real complaints or rumors based on anecdotes. Note that if the company becomes aware of a publication, such as a letter-to-the-editor of a medical journal or a newspaper report, that describes a death, injury, or safety hazard related to one of its devices, the company should treat this as a complaint and act upon it.

❖ The names and signatures of those who performed the initial review of the complaint, and the dates of their review.

❖ The names of the individuals and units responsible for the final resolution of the complaint, and the date the report was transmitted to them.

96. **The Complaint Closure Report.** This should be placed in the same file folder or document class as the original complaint report. All complaints should be closed out with a closure report. Even complaints that were not investigated need to attain closure, since a decision not to take action is, in itself, an action.

The closure report should contain the information requested in 21 CFR 820.198(e)(6)–(8) and a discussion of the points mentioned in 21 CFR 820.198(d). In addition to the regulatory requirements, the following information should be included in the closure report.

❖ Any additional information that was obtained as a result of the investigation of the complaint. This should include any additional details obtained from the complainant as well as the results of any testing performed by the company.

❖ Corrective action requests and corrective actions that resulted from the investigation of the complaint. Note that the complaint cannot come to closure until all corrective action requests associated with the complaint have also been closed.

❖ The names and departments of all individuals who were involved in responding to the complaint, along with their memberships in corrective action teams, auditing teams, special troubleshooting teams, or other working groups.

❖ If possible, keep records of all communications between the company and the complainant. If the investigation was large and complex, it will be useful to obtain a letter or other statement from the complainant, indicating the person's level of satisfaction with the response and whether or not additional information or help is needed.

❖ The names and signatures of the individuals who were responsible for investigating and responding to the complaint. They should also be able to make the statement that the complaint was closed to the satisfaction of the company and there were no known outstanding issues at the time of closure.

The response or report to regulatory agencies should be transmitted through the company's regulatory affairs unit, who should review and approve the response before transmission. The response to the complainant should be passed through the customer service unit, who should review the response before transmission to the complainant. In both cases, the response must be checked for potential legal consequences before transmission.

97. **Location.** The location of the complaint unit and complaint records should be specified. If the complaint unit is separate from the manufacturing location, a document needs to be written to instruct the complaint handling unit to ensure the copying of all complaint records and placement of these copies at a specified location in the device's manufacturing plant. The responsibility for maintaining the complaint files at the manufacturing location should also be specified. Regardless of how a complaint is received, there must be a mechanism that ensures the placement of copies of the complaint report with both the complaint unit and with the unit that actually manufactures the device.

   If the manufacturer's complaint unit or the manufacturer itself is located outside of the United States, a document needs to be prepared specifying a location within the United States as a repository for copies of complaint files. As in the case of the company with separate manufacturing and complaint handling locations, this document should specify locations and responsibilities for maintaining current copies of complaints. This U.S. location might be a company subsidiary or an agent contracted to act as a complaint handling unit.

❄ Subpart N—Servicing ❄

21 CFR 820.200 Servicing

(a) Where servicing is a specified requirement, each manufacturer shall establish and maintain instructions and procedures for performing and verifying that the servicing meets the specified requirements.

(b) Each manufacturer shall analyze service reports with appropriate statistical methodology in accordance with Sec. 820.100.

(c) Each manufacturer who receives a service report that represents an event which must be reported to FDA under part 803 or 804 of this chapter shall automatically consider the report a complaint and shall process it in accordance with the requirements of Sec. 820.198.

(d) Service reports shall be documented and shall include:

(1) The name of the device serviced;
(2) Any device identification(s) and control number(s) used;
(3) The date of service;
(4) The individual(s) servicing the device;
(5) The service performed; and
(6) The test and inspection data.

98. **Service Manual.** The manufacturer can ignore paragraph 21 CFR 820.200, if the device being manufactured does not or cannot require servicing. These would be items such as single use devices that are discarded or destroyed during or after use, or devices that are so inexpensive that an occasional defective unit would be discarded rather than being rebuilt or repaired. In all other cases, the manufacturer (or refurbisher) will need to prepare a service or maintenance manual that will be used by personnel who will maintain or repair the device after it is released for distribution. All servicing whether performed by the manufacturer or a third party needs to meet the requirements of this regulation.

While the service or maintenance manual will, naturally, need to contain instructions on how to service or repair the device. It will also need to contain instructions on how to test the device after servicing to measure parameters that will show that the serviced device will meet the original criteria, demonstrating its ability to operate in a safe and effective manner. The acceptance limits for these parameters should be stated in the manual and, if necessary, affixed to the machine. Handling instructions to meet the needs of 21 CFR 820.140 should be included in the manual. All servicing-related documents, especially those related to servicing methods and procedures, should become a part of the DMR.

The service or maintenance manual should also contain instructions to the servicing personnel to direct the person receiving the request for servicing to ascertain the reasons for the service request. This person should be trained in the reporting requirements of 21 CFR 803 and 21 CFR 804, so that they would be able to act upon any need for immediate reporting of a serious patient-related event. The requirements for 21 CFR 803 should be discussed along with the regulations in 21 CFR 820.198. Because of the usual lag time between a service request and the actual service, it is important that the people who receive the requests be trained to assess the possibility that the service request really represents a situation that is covered under 21 CFR 803.

A problem arises if the device is relatively easy to service or repair. Unlike a complex device that could be serviced by only the original manufacturer or specialized shops known to the manufacturer, this type of device may attract shops who are unknown to the manufacturer and whose activities and general behavior are completely out of the control of the original manufacturer. Although all servicing must be performed in accordance with these regulations, these shops may not understand reporting requirements or operate under any GMP rules at all. The manufacturer must take steps to control and prevent this type of activity. Warning the customer and providing a list of service centers or cooperative servicing shops might be a step to take. A clear statement of requirements in the service manual and a label attached to the device would also be useful.

The service manual must be available to servicing shops who are independent from the manufacturer. This must be done to ensure the proper servicing of the device even when performed by an independent firm. Third party servicers must perform the service according to the manufacturer's instructions and maintain records of the servicing just as though they were affiliated with the manufacturer. Third party servicers are also required to provide copies of the service reports described in 21 CFR 820.200(d) to the manufacturer. The manufacturer should include these instructions in the servicing manual in a prominent format to aid in informing independent servicers of their responsibilities.

99. **Service Reports.** A document should be prepared to cover service reports and their handling. The service report should contain the information required in 21 CFR 820.200(d)(1)–(6) and additional information. The additional information would be the reason for the service work; the circumstances that led to the request for service; the information generated during the evaluation of the serviced device, including the results of any tests; and a brief evaluation of the device's fitness-for-use. The signature of the person providing the service is not required by the regulation but would be useful for auditing purposes. The information contained in the report should show the device's status with regard to safety and fitness-for-use and support the evaluation given by the service provider. It will also be useful to provide a clear indicator on the device to show its servicing status, particularly with respect to meeting basic requirements for functionality.

A good approach would be to have this document create a service report template that would contain blanks, check-off boxes, and comment spaces. This template could be placed in the service and repair manual and photocopies made as needed. The template would be accompanied by instructions on how to fill it out, and the distribution of copies. One copy should be retained by the service provider or the servicing organization. One copy should be sent to a group that will be in a position to evaluate all of the service reports to determine any need for corrective or preventive action. Trending and other statistical analyses should be performed following the procedures given under 21 CFR 820.250. Even if there is no complaint of such a severity as to require action under 21 CFR 820.198, if quality related trends, potential hazards, or systemic problems are found, they should be treated as requiring corrective action under the provisions of 21 CFR 820.100, and if necessary, the group reviewing the service reports should issue a corrective action request. Each service report should be treated as having the potential to result in a corrective action. The evaluating group should be charged with the responsibilities related to 21 CFR 820.100, but groups dealing with acceptance status (21 CFR 820.80 and 21 CFR 820.86) or nonconforming product (21 CFR 820.90) might also be employed if they are assigned the responsibility. Finally, one copy should go into the device history record for the device or lot of devices.

With a device that may require servicing, there is a need to be able to identify the exact device that was serviced or refurbished. For this reason, the procedures under 21 CFR 820.60 and 21 CFR 820.65 may be very useful, even if they are not specifically required for a particular device. Only a totally harmless device, as demonstrated by a risk analysis, does not need identification and traceability. In all other cases, it may be important to know if repair or servicing may have been related to a serious event, and only a good tracing system will allow the manufacturer to determine the situation with regard to the injury-causing device.

❈ Subpart O— ❈
Statistical Techniques

21 CFR 820.250 Statistical Techniques

21 CFR 820.250(a) *Where appropriate, each manufacturer shall establish and maintain procedures for identifying valid statistical techniques required for establishing, controlling, and verifying the acceptability of process capability and product characteristics.*
21 CFR 820.250(b) *Sampling plans, when used, shall be written and based on a valid statistical rationale. Each manufacturer shall*

establish and maintain procedures to ensure that sampling methods are adequate for their intended use and to ensure that when changes occur the sampling plans are reviewed. These activities shall be documented.

100. **Statistical Manual.** This section on statistical techniques basically requires the preparation of a statistical manual for the company. While the regulation says that this needs to be done only where appropriate, just about any company that produces large quantities of products can benefit from having proper statistical methods to monitor and evaluate its activities. The statistical manual should be prepared even if the company has one or more statisticians. In statistics, there is often more than one way to approach a problem or to test a hypothesis. It is important for a manufacturer to have uniform procedures throughout the different departments and divisions, and this manual will help to develop that uniformity. Also, as personnel change, the statistical manual will maintain continuity in the company's procedures. At the present stage of the regulations, the manual should consist of three major sections to cover each of the areas mentioned in 21 CFR 820.250.

In addition to this manual, the company should purchase a well-written textbook on statistical procedures and make it available for use by personnel who need to be trained in statistical methods. This book should be established as the company reference to minimize conflicts arising from the use of different texts. A good statistical software package or a spreadsheet package with useful statistical functions should also be obtained and established. The effective use of statistical procedures usually requires a large amount of data processing, so a good software package will be of great help. Do not purchase texts or software that are primarily useful to professional statisticians. The material must be usable in the laboratory and on the manufacturing floor by nonstatisticians. The document needed here should establish the statistical manual, references, and the general system for collecting, reviewing, and processing statistical data. As with any procedural documents that involve numerical manipulations, examples should be provided for the readers.

101. **Statistical Process Control.** Process capability can be evaluated by Statistical Process Control (SPC). SPC, if used, must be performed at the level of the operator or line worker. The documents for SPC must be prepared in a manner that is intelligible to these workers, who may not be well-grounded in algebra. There are several good manuals covering SPC, and training courses are offered by several organizations. The American Society for Quality Certified Quality Engineers (CQEs) are trained in the use of SPC and other statistical procedures useful for general manufacturing and monitoring. Under the guidance of an individual trained in the use of SPC, the manufacturer should prepare an SPC manual that is tailored for the company's operations. This manual will be the document needed here. SPC can be used for processes other than manufacturing. Processes, such as receiving, servicing, and complaint reporting, may also be monitored by this method. The SPC document should define what constitutes a controlled process for the various steps in the manufacturing of the device. Actions to be taken when a process goes out of control should also be specified.

102. **Sampling Procedures.** Procedures for drawing random samples from a lot of many units need to be defined. The simple first, middle, and last, method is not always the best. The basic requirements here is that any sampling plan needs to be justified. There are times when nonrandom sampling is best, especially for checking the worst case, and this will require justification. Many companies have adopted Military Standards 105E and 414 (Recently reissued as ANSI/ASQ documents) and their relatives for attribute and variable testing. These procedures and their associated tables should be incorporated into the sampling procedures manual along with solved examples based on actual manufacturing data. Even if the manufacturer does not currently plan to use statistical sampling procedures, it is a good idea to obtain copies of the Standards to have them available for use, if needed. Once again, a certified quality engineer could prove useful to a manufacturer.

103. **General Procedures.** The final part will cover general statistical procedures of the type that are used to study laboratory

test data and look for differences between groups of data. It should cover basic procedures, such as calculating means, variances, standard deviations, coefficients of variation, the 95% confidence interval about the mean, the t-test, and the F-ratio. Linear regression and simple analysis of variance should also be covered. Trending should be discussed, along with the methods to use in order to detect trends. Examples should be worked out not only to show how the procedures work, but also to provide examples of how the procedures should be employed in day-to-day work.

It will be helpful if this document could also cover the abuse of statistics and define practices that should be avoided. Averaging to conceal an out-of-specification result and conditions that result in a breakdown of the normal distribution assumption should be covered. The subject of data recording and the requirement that all data, not just averages, must be recorded could also be discussed here.

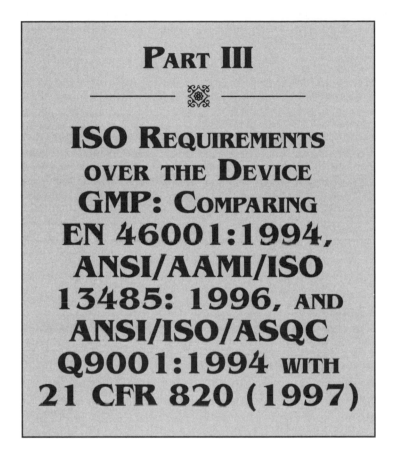

PART III

ISO REQUIREMENTS OVER THE DEVICE GMP: COMPARING EN 46001:1994, ANSI/AAMI/ISO 13485: 1996, AND ANSI/ISO/ASQC Q9001:1994 WITH 21 CFR 820 (1997)

This section relates 21 CFR 820 (1997) requirements to ANSI/ISO/ASQC 9001:1994, ANSI/AAMI/ISO 13485:1996, and EN 46001:1994 with the idea of providing a guide to meeting ANSI/ISO/ASQC 9001:1994 requirements. This guide is based on the idea that a manufacturer will already be in the process of complying with the CGMP and needs to know what additional documents will be needed for ANSI/ISO/ASQC 9001 compliance. If no comments are made in the tables that follow, the author feels that the ISO item in the left column, and any associated ANSI/AAMI/ISO 13485 or EN 46001:1994 section, is met by compliance with the Device CGMP item in the right column. Where the Device CGMP section will not cover the requirement in the ISO section, or if the coverage is incomplete, a discussion is provided on how the ANSI/ISO/ASQC 9001:1994, ANSI/AAMI/ISO 13485:1996, or EN 46001 requirements can be met. In some or most instances, it is possible to argue that an ISO requirement that is supposedly not covered by the Device CGMP, is really covered if a Device CGMP paragraph is interpreted in a certain manner. The author prefers a more direct route that does not depend on interpretations that may or may not find acceptance by particular inspectors or auditors.

When comparing ISO and Quality System regulations, the reader should be aware of a major qualitative difference that exists between these two sets of standards. An ISO audit is conducted with the ultimate goal of helping to strengthen the auditee's quality system and to verify the auditee's conformance with ISO standards. The auditor is, ultimately, an employee of the auditee and has authority only to the extent created by the auditee's need to gain or maintain ISO certification. A U.S. auditee may decide to ignore the audit findings and decide not to seek an ISO certification or to give up a current registration. An FDA inspection is not a quality audit in the usual sense. The FDA inspector is a federal employee who is there to assess compliance with federal regulations, which have the status of law. The FDA inspector is acting to protect the consumer and not just assessing the manufacturer's ability to satisfy quality system requirements. The company being inspected cannot ignore the findings of an FDA inspection, at least if they wish to remain in business, and civil or criminal litigation against the company or individuals within the company may arise from inspections that reveal serious or repeated violations. Consequently, FDA regulations are just that, regulations, while ISO standards are more like guidelines where voluntary compliance is possible. If a company cannot meet ISO standards, it can continue to do business, at least in the United States, but a company that does not meet FDA regulations will be unable to market its products.

The point is that FDA regulations must be followed by all U.S.-based device manufacturers who wish to do business in the medical area. Thus, the regulations that are found in 21 CFR 820 are a basic part of the cost of doing business in the United States, but compliance with ISO regulations may be regarded as a source of additional costs that do not need to be borne by a U.S. manufacturer. On the other hand, there are many geographic locations where FDA regulations do not apply, and compliance with the more universal ISO standards will provide a company with regulatory and marketing advantages. The recent efforts at tripartite harmonization of requirements among the United States, Japan, and the European Union have brought FDA and ISO requirements, in the device area at least, closer together. The question then becomes, "What more does a company need to do to comply with ANSI/ISO/ASQC 9001 if it is already complying with FDA regulations?" As will be seen below, the additional work is really not that great. ISO compliance may only require a few new documents and minor modifications to already existing documents. The next question is then one of what and where? The discussion in this part is designed to answer this question. Remember that ANSI/ISO/ASQC 9001, 9002, and 9003 are basically the same standards with portions removed from 9001 (design control for instance) to create 9002 and 9003. Thus, the discussion of ANSI/ISO/ASQC 9001 can be made into a discussion of 9002 or 9003 by ignoring appropriate sections.

For certain medical devices there are other, European, documents that should be obtained and reviewed. These documents are based on ANSI/ISO/ASQC 9001 and contain more specific instructions on how compliance with the ANSI/ISO/ASQC 9001 is to be accomplished. These documents are specifically applicable for European nations that are members of the European Committee for Standardization (CEN) and the European Committee for Electrotechnical Standardization (CENELEC), who jointly issued these standards via the Joint CEN/CENELEC Coordinated Working Group on Quality Supplements. Copies of these standards in English may be obtained from the British Standards Institute (BSI) or their agents such as the American National Standards Institute (ANSI). The first document, which is also the more comprehensive, is EN 46001:1994, "Specification for Application of EN 29001 (BS 5750 : Part 1) to the Manufacture of Medical Devices." (Note that BS 5750:Part 1 is the same as EN 29001 which, in turn, is the same as ANSI/ISO/ASQC 9001.) Another important document is ANSI/AAMI/ISO 13485:1996, "Quality

Systems—Medical Devices—Supplementary requirements to ISO 9001." The other documents are prEN 50103 "Guidance on the application of EN 29001 and EN 46001 and EN 29002 and EN 46002 for the active (including active implantable) medical device industry," and prEN 724 "Guidance on the Application of EN 29001 and EN 46001 and of EN 29002 and EN 46002 for non-active medical devices." In this book, ANSI/AAMI/ISO 13485:1996 and EN 46001 have been reviewed and are discussed where applicable, but neither prEN 724 nor prEN 50103 have been considered, because they were considered to be specialized to particular types of devices.

The manufacturer should note that compliance with ANSI/ ISO/ASQC 9000 standards may not be sufficient for a particular medical device. If the manufacturer will be seeking the CE Mark in Europe, there are other requirements that must be met, based on the Medical Device Directive, and additional standards or regulations will need to be reviewed. If the manufacturer will be seeking Underwriters Laboratories (UL) or Canadian Standards Association (CSA) certifications or ratings, there will be a need for additional testing and procedures. In addition, there may be other regional certifying bodies whose requirements may need to be met. In general, compliance with the ANSI/ISO/ASQC 9000 standards should help a company to gain the other certifications, but it is no guarantee of acceptance.

After the preceding paragraph, the reader is probably beginning to suspect that there are many more applicable documents than just those related to the ANSI/ISO/ASQC 9000 series. There are thousands of ISO standards that apply to many different areas. There is an amazing proliferation of standards and guidelines, which are distributed through only a few sources at a cost that usually precludes the purchase of personal copies. In general, English language versions of European standards can be obtained through British organizations. If the manufacturer does not have a full-time Regulatory Affairs staff, the services of a consultant will be valuable. In this book, only the ISO documents that relate to quality systems will be covered. Even among these documents there is a large variety of standards and guidelines, so some selection, concentrating on medical device-related subjects, has been done.

First of all, in order to use the ANSI/ISO/ASQC 9001 series, the manufacturer should obtain copies of ISO 9000-1 and 9000-2, which are general guidelines for the application of ANSI/ISO/ASQC 9001, 9002, and 9003. ISO 9004-4, 10005, and 10006 provide general quality assurance guidelines. In addition to these, ISO 9004-1 provides guidelines for quality management and quality systems, as does ISO 10002. Both of these provide useful guidance when considering parts 4.1 and 4.2 of ANSI/ISO/ASQC 9001. ISO 10013, the guideline for quality manuals, is discussed later in this text, as is the standard for definitions known as, ANSI/ISO/ASQC A8402:1994, "Quality Management and Quality Assurance—Vocabulary." This was approved as an American National Standard on February 6, 1995, and many definitions now used with 21 CFR 820 were derived from it. Also, ANSI/AAMI/ISO 13485:1996 and EN 46001 were produced with the aim of providing supplemental regulations to help the medical device manufacturer meet the requirements of ANSI/ISO/ASQC 9001. It appears that ANSI/AAMI/ISO 13485, which is a international standard, will eventually replace EN 46001 which was a standard only for the European community.

Other useful guidelines are ISO 9000-3 for software, 9000-4 for dependability management, 9004-3 for processed materials, 10015 for education and training, and 10016 for presenting inspection and test results. Quality auditing is covered in ISO 10011 in three parts, and the quality assurance of measuring equipment is covered in two parts in ISO 10012. While these documents are primarily aimed at helping the manufacturer to comply with ISO standards, they are also useful when working with the CGMPs. They will often provide useful insights into procedures for complying with the corresponding parts of 21 CFR 820, and they are especially useful if the manufacturer ultimately will be seeking ISO registration.

※ Tables ※

In the following tables, numbers in the left column refer to paragraphs that will be found in ANSI/ISO/ASQC 9001:1994. Numbers in the right column refer to parts and paragraphs in the Quality System regulations (Device GMP requirements) given in 21 CFR 820. The left column lists the requirements of the ANSI/ISO/ASQC 9001:1994 standard, and the right column lists that portion of the Quality System regulations (21 CFR 820) that should meet the requirements of the ANSI/ISO/ASQC standard. The purpose here is to show how the Quality System regulations will meet the needs of the ISO standards and indicate the areas where the two standards are not complementary, and the Quality System regulations do not meet the needs of the ISO standard. In these situations, additional documents or additions to existing documents may be required to meet the ISO standard.

When reviewing the contents of this table and the discussion in the following section, the reader should refer to ANSI/ISO/ASQC A8402:1994 and Part 3 of ANSI/AAMI/ISO 13485 for the definitions of key terms.

ANSI/ISO/ASQC 9001:1994	21 CFR 820 (Quality System regulations)
4. Quality Systems Requirements	820.1(a)(1) with a definition in 820.3(v) and a description in Subpart B.
4.1 Management Responsibility 4.1.1 Quality Policy	820.20 (a) and 820.186 for documentation and a definition in 820.3(u).
4.1.2 Organization	820.20 (b)
4.1.2.1 Responsibility and Authority 4.1.2.1a) Prevent the Occurrence of Nonconformities 4.1.2.1b) Identify and Record Problems 4.1.2.1c) Provide Solutions 4.1.2.1d) Verify Implementation 4.1.2.1e) Control Further Processing	820.20 (b)(1) 820.20 (b)(1) and the definition in 820.3(aa).
4.1.2.2 Resources for Quality	820.20 (b)(2)
4.1.2.3 Management Representative	820.20 (b)(3) and the definition in 820.3(n).
4.1.2.3a) Quality System Establishment	820.20 (e)

ANSI/ISO/ASQC 9001:1994	21 CFR 820 (Quality System regulations)
4.1.2.3b) Quality System Performance Reporting	820.20 (b)(3)(ii)
4.1.3 Management Review	820.20 (c)
4.2 Quality System	820.3(v) gives a definition. Instructions to manufacturers are given in 820.5 and 820.20(e) requires an outline of the structure of the quality and documentation system.
4.2.1 General States that a Quality Manual (QM) shall be prepared that will include or make reference to the procedures and regulations used in the Quality System. The preparation of a QM is not covered in 21 CFR 820.	
4.2.2 Quality System Procedures Mainly concerned with the idea that procedures will be documented and implemented.	820.5 and 820.20(e) mainly require the documentation of quality system procedures. The implication, of course, is that they will be implemented as well.
4.2.3 Quality Planning The full ANSI/ISO/ASQC 9001 should be reviewed to ensure the complete coverage of this section.	820.3(u), 820.5 and 820.20(d). Parts 4.2.3a) and 4.2.3h) are covered by the CFR sections, but other parts may require additional details. Quality planning should be included in the activities covered by 820.30 and run in parallel with design planning.
4.2.3a) Preparation of Quality Plans	820.20(d) and 820.30
4.2.3c) Compatibility of Design	820.30(b), (d), (e), (f), and (g)
4.2.3f) Identification of Verification	820.30(f) and 820.70 (a)
4.2.3g) Standards of Acceptability	820.30(d) and (f), 820.70 (a), and 820.80
4.2.3h) Identification and Preparation of Quality Records	820.20(e), 820.181, and 820.186

ANSI/ISO/ASQC 9001:1994	21 CFR 820 (Quality System regulations)
4.3 Contract Review 4.3.1 General	820.50 and 820.160
4.3.2a) Definition of Requirements	820.50 (b)
4.3.2b) Resolution of Differences Covered only by implication in 820.50 for purchased material but is covered in 820.160 for devices that are sold.	
4.3.2c) Capability of Meeting Requirements Refers to the ability of the supplier (manufacturer) to meet contractual obligations imposed by the purchaser of the supplier's product. It does not appear that 21 CFR 820 covers this subject.	
4.3.3 Amendment to Contract Requires the manufacturer to identify how a contract amendment is made and the information correctly transferred to the concerned functions within the manufacturer's organization.	
4.3.4 Records of Contract Reviews	820.160

ANSI/ISO/ASQC 9001:1994	21 CFR 820 (Quality System regulations)
4.4 Design Control 4.4.1 General	820.30 (a). The device classification given here does not exist in the ANSI/ISO/ASQC 9001, EN 46001, or ANSI/AAMI/ISO 13485:1996.
4.4.2 Design and Development Planning	820.30 (b)
4.4.3 Organizational and Technical Interfaces	820.30 (b)
4.4.4 Design Input	820.3(f) gives a definition, 820.30 (a) and (c)
4.4.5 Design Output Refers to identifying characteristics crucial to the safe and proper functioning of the product. The term "safe" is not included in 820.30 (d).	820.3(g) gives a definition, 820.30(d). The need for "safe functioning" is implied in the requirement for "proper functioning" and in the guideline on "Do It by Design."
4.4.6 Design Review	820.3(h) contains a definition, 820.30 (e)
4.4.7 Design Verification ANSI/AAMI/ISO 13485:1996 requires the documentation of clinical investigations and risk analyses related to design verification.	820.30(f). For guidance on risk analysis, see ISO/CD 14971, "Medical Devices—Risk Management—Application of Risk Analysis to Medical Devices."
4.4.8 Design Validation ANSI/AAMI/ISO 13485:1996 requires the documentation of clinical investigations and risk analyses related to design validation.	820.30(f), (g), and (h)
4.4.9 Design Changes	820.30(i)
4.5 Document and Data Control 4.5.1 General	820.40
4.5.2 Document & Data Approval & Issue In 4.5.2c) the ISO standard requires the identification of obsolete documents that are retained for legal or other purposes.	820.40(a)
4.5.3 Document and Data Changes	820.40(b)

ANSI/ISO/ASQC 9001:1994	21 CFR 820 (Quality System regulations)
4.6 Purchasing 4.6.1 General	820.50
4.6.2 Evaluation of Subcontractors	820.50(a)
4.6.3 Purchasing Data Contains specific requirements that are not necessarily the same as the requirements for 820.50(b).	820.50(b)
4.6.4 Verification of Purchased Product 4.6.4.1 Refers to the supplier (manufacturer) performing verification activities at the subcontractor's premises. 4.6.4.2 Refers to the supplier's (manufacturer's) customer or customer's representative conducting verification activities at the subcontractor's premises.	820.80(a) and (b) contain general requirements for the verification of purchased products with no reference to the location at which these activities may take place.
4.7 Control of Customer-Supplied Product Contains a requirement for controlling any maintenance of customer-supplier product and for notifying the customer of any lost or unusable product.	820.80(a) and (b) deal with the acceptance and verification of incoming product, and 820.150 covers the storage of all products. Customer-supplied product is treated like any other incoming product.
4.8 Product Identification and Traceability Some differences are found in EN 46001.	820.60, 820.65, 820.90(a), 820.160, and 820.200. For tracked devices, see 21 CFR 821.
4.9 Process Control EN 46001 contains material discussed later.	820.70(a), 820.75, 820.170, and 820.200
4.9a) Documented Procedures	820.70(a) and (c), 820.75, 820.170, and 820.200
4.9b) Suitable Equipment and Environment	820.70(a), (c), (f) and (g), 820.170, and 820.200
4.9c) Compliance	820.70(a)(1) and (3)
4.9d) Monitoring and Control	820.70(a)(2)

ANSI/ISO/ASQC 9001:1994	21 CFR 820 (Quality System regulations)
4.9e) Approvals of Processes and Equipment	820.70(a)(4)
4.9f) Criteria for Workmanship	820.70(a)(5)
4.9g) Equipment Maintenance	820.70(g)
4.10 Inspection and Testing 4.10.1 General	820.80(a)
4.10.2 Receiving Inspection and Testing 4.10.2.1 Incoming Product	820.80(b)
4.10.2.2 Control at Subcontractor's Premises	Other than general requirements, the Device CGMPs do not suggest giving considerations based on the amount of control exercised at the subcontractor's premises.
4.10.2.3 Release for Urgent Purposes	820.80(d) Other than requiring that final product shall not be released for distribution until all activities required by the Device Master Record have been completed, the Device CGMP does not directly address the handling of product that is released prior to the completion of verification activities.
4.10.3 In-process Inspection and Testing	820.80(c)
4.10.4 Final Inspection and Testing	820.80(d)
4.10.5 Inspection and Test Records	820.80(d) and (e) and 820.180

ANSI/ISO/ASQC 9001:1994	21 CFR 820 (Quality System regulations)
4.11 Control of Inspection, Measuring, and Test Equipment 4.11.1 General	820.72
4.11.2a) Selecting Measurements and Criteria Requires the determination of the measurements to be made, the accuracy required, and a selection of appropriate test equipment that can provide the needed accuracy and precision.	820.72(b)
4.11.2b) Identify and Calibrate Equipment	820.72(a) and (b)
4.11.2c) Calibration Process	820.72(b)
4.11.2d) Calibration Status Identification	820.72(b)(2)
4.11.2e) Maintain Calibration Records	820.72(b)(2)
4.11.2f) Validity of Previous Results Requires a review of previous inspection and test results when test equipment is found to be out of calibration.	
4.11.2g) Suitable Environmental Conditions Requires suitable environmental conditions for the activities being conducted with the test and measurement equipment.	820.72(a) Provides for the handling, preservation, and storage of test equipment to maintain fitness-for-use. Other than requiring that the equipment be capable of producing valid results, 820.72 does not address the operating environment.
4.11.2h) Handling, etc. of Test Equipment	820.72(a)
4.11.2i) Safeguard from Adjustments that May Invalidate Calibrations	820.72(a)
4.12 Inspection and Test Status	820.86

ANSI/ISO/ASQC 9001:1994	21 CFR 820 (Quality System regulations)
4.13 Control of Nonconforming Product 4.13.1 General	820.3(q) and 820.90(a) and (b)
4.13.2 Review and Disposition Contains four methods for the disposition of nonconforming product.	820.90(b)
4.14 Corrective and Preventive Action 4.14.1 General	820.100
4.14.2 Corrective Action Procedures ANSI/AAMI/ISO 13485:1996 supplements ANSI/ISO/ASQC 9001. 4.14.2a) Handling of Customer Complaints	820.3(b), 820.100(a)(1), and 820.198
4.14.2b) Investigation of Nonconformities	820.90(b) and 820.100(a)(2)
4.14.2c) Determination of Corrective Action Needed	820.100(a)(3)
4.14.2d) Controlling Corrective Action	820.100(a)(4) and (5)
4.14.3 Preventive Action	820.100(a)(4), (6), (7), 820.198(e), and 820.200(b)
4.15 Handling, Storage, Packaging, Preservation, and Delivery 4.15.1 General	820.130, 820.140, 820.150, and 820.160
4.15.2 Handling	820.140
4.15.3 Storage	820.150

ISO 9001:1994	21 CFR 820 (Quality System regulations)
4.15.4 Packaging Refers to "marking" that will be covered under 820.120 if the marking constitutes labeling. ANSI/AAMI/ISO 13485:1996 defines marking as labeling.	820.120 and 820.130
4.15.5 Preservation	820.120(c) and 820.150
4.15.6 Delivery Requires protection of product quality after final inspection, including, where specified, delivery to its destination.	820.160 requires control and distribution of finished devices to ensure that only approved devices are released. Also see 21 CFR 821 for tracked devices.
4.16 Control of Quality Records Contains a specific requirement for documenting procedures for the identification, collection, indexing, access, filing, storage, maintenance, and disposition of quality records, including quality records from subcontractors.	820.186 and 820.180 in part
4.17 Internal Quality Audits	820.3(t) and 820.22
4.18 Training	820.25(a) and (b)
4.19 Servicing	820.200
4.20 Statistical Techniques	820.250

※ Additional Documents or ※ Considerations Needed to Meet ANSI/ISO/ASQC 9001:1994, ANSI/AAMI/ISO 13485:1996, and EN 46001:1994 Requirements

The following discussions, which are about any additional documents necessary to meet the requirements of ANSI/ISO/ASQC 9001:1994, ANSI/AAMI/ISO 13485:1996, and EN 46001:1994, are listed by ANSI/ISO/ASQC 9001 sections or paragraphs. When a section or paragraph is not mentioned, it may be assumed that the corresponding requirements of 21 CFR 820 will meet the requirements of the section from ANSI/ISO/ASQC 9001. The following section covers only those situations where it is felt that the Quality System regulation does not satisfy the requirements of the section from the ANSI/ISO/ASQC standard. The reader is urged to obtain a current copy of ANSI/ISO/ASQC 9001:1994 and to review pertinent sections. The reader should also obtain current copies of ANSI/AAMI/ISO 13485:1996, and EN 46001:1994. Note that EN 29001 is the same as ANSI/ISO/ASQC 9001, except that the EN series represents European Standards. Readers in certain segments of the medical device industry may also wish to obtain copies of prEN 50103, "Guidance on the application of EN 29001 and EN 46001 and EN 29002 and EN 46002 for the active (including active implantable) medical device industry," prEN 724 "Guidance on the application of quality systems for the non-active medical device industry," or prEN 928 "Guidance on the application of EN 29001/EN 46001 and EN 29002/EN 46002 for the in vitro diagnostic industry." The equivalence or nonequivalence of sections of the CFR and ISO (including EN 46001 and ANSI/AAMI/ISO 13485:1996) requirements are based on the author's experience and interpretations and the reader may want a more specific review that covers the situation for the reader's firm, rather than accept the author's generalizations.

For those sections that are not completely covered by the GMPs, the discussion will start with a quotation, in italics, of the appropriate ANSI/ISO/ASQC 9001:1994 section. Comments based on EN 46001 or ANSI/AAMI/ISO 13485:1996 alone will also be made, but these comments will not be quotations. The reader should assume that the ANSI/AAMI/ISO 13485:1996 and EN 46001 sections correspond to the ANSI/ISO/ASQC 9001 sections, unless otherwise noted. These quotations will then be followed by the author's comments and recommendations, if any. Remember that in ISO documents the "supplier" is the same as the "manufacturer" in CGMP regulations, and the vendor who sells to the manufacturer is often known as the subcontractor. For definitions refer to Section 1 of ANSI/ISO/ASQC A8402:1994. The manufacturer should have a copy of this document since it has been adopted as an American National Standard.

※ ANSI/ISO/ASQC 9001:1994 ※ Part 4. Quality Systems Requirements

4.1 Management Responsibility

4.1.2 Organization

4.1.2.1 Responsibility and Authority. *The responsibility, authority, and the interrelation of personnel who manage, perform, and verify work affecting quality shall be defined and documented, particularly for personnel who need the organizational freedom and authority to:*

4.1.2.1a) *Initiate action to prevent the occurrence of any nonconformities relating to product, process, and quality system;*

4.1.2.1b) *Identify and record any problems relating to the product, process, and quality system;*

4.1.2.1c) *Initiate, recommend or provide solutions through designated channels;*

4.1.2.1e) (Note that 4.1.2.1d) is addressed elsewhere.) *Control further processing, delivery, or installation of nonconforming product until the deficiency or unsatisfactory condition has been corrected.*

A document or part of a document should delineate the responsibility, authority, and working interrelationships of personnel who are responsible for the actions noted in paragraphs a, b, c, and e above. These might be added to documents prepared in support of 21 CFR

820.20(b)(1) and (2). The company is expected to describe and document its quality system, and it should be a relatively simple matter to specifically address these activities in documents that need to be prepared anyway. Statements concerning the movement of nonconforming product during processing, delivery, or installation should be inserted into documents concerning these activities (See 21 CFR 820.90(a)). If all employees are empowered to prevent or eliminate nonconformities, this should be expressed in a high level document, such as one that is in the Quality Manual. In general, it would seem that these responsibilities should either be assigned to all personnel or restricted to a specific group.

It is very important that all employees understand their responsibilities for quality and the authority that they have for meeting these responsibilities. An organizational chart showing positions and their relationships, coupled with a table of responsibilities and appropriate specific job descriptions, would go far toward addressing the above requirements. The reader should note that diffuse and generalized assignments of responsibilities and authority usually result in generalized indifference and nonacceptance of responsibility.

4.2 Quality System

4.2.1 General. *The supplier shall establish, document, and maintain a quality system as a means of ensuring that product conforms to specified requirements. The supplier shall prepare a quality manual covering the requirements of this American National Standard. The quality manual shall include or make reference to the quality system procedures and outline the structure of the documentation used in the quality system.*

Note 6 *Guidance on quality manuals is given in ISO 10013.*

The difference between this part and the corresponding paragraph in 21 CFR 820 lies in the ISO requirement that a firm should document its quality system by means of a Quality Manual (QM). In general, the QM is a collection of high level documents that describe how the company is addressing the different elements of ANSI/ISO/ASQC 9001:1994 and usually constitutes the top tier in the hierarchy of quality related documents. Specific functional responsibilities and work instructions (SOPs, runsheets, travelers) are usually covered in lower level documents. Because of the variety of approaches that may be used for preparing and maintaining a QM, the standard known as ISO 10013 "Guidelines for Developing Quality Manuals" should be consulted. Both ISO standards and 21 CFR 820 regulations require the preparation of an outline of the structure of the documentation system. It is best if the preparation of the QM and this outline were done together.

EN 46001:1994 requires the supplier to establish and document the specified requirements of the quality system. The supplier is expected to maintain a file that contains the product, manufacturing, and quality assurance specifications for each type or model of medical device that is manufactured. If a file is not maintained, the location of the information must be given. This requirement should be met by conformance with 21 CFR 820.181, which covers the Device Master Record.

4.2.3 Quality Planning. *The supplier shall define and document how the requirements for quality will be met. Quality planning shall be consistent with all other requirements of a supplier's quality system and shall be documented in a format to suit the supplier's method of operation. The supplier shall give consideration to the following activities, as appropriate, in meeting the specified requirements for products, projects, or contracts:*

Note 8 *The quality plans referred to (see 4.2.3a) may be in the form of a reference to the appropriate documented procedures that form an integral part of the supplier's quality system.*

Subparagraphs a, c, f, and h of this part are covered by the cited sections of 21 CFR 820, but other parts appear to need additional documentation. The quality planning section relates to the manufacturer's quality planning in regard to the requirements for the manufacturer's products, projects, or contracts. The ISO standard states that the manufacturer will document quality planning and give appropriate consideration to subparagraphs b, d, and f, below. This quality planning should go beyond the requirements for design planning. The requirements of ANSI/AAMI/ISO 13485 can be met with the DMR (21 CFR 820.18) and the quality systems records (21 CFR 820.186).

4.2.3b) *The identification and acquisition of any controls, processes, equipment (including inspection and test equipment), fixtures, resources, and skills that may be needed to achieve the required quality;*

This requirement in 4.2.3b) can be met at the product development stage by including quality planning as part of the product development or design development process. The quality planning should become a part of project management and be documented as such. A "quality requirements" document could be prepared to address the concerns of this part.

In the case of existing products, a "quality review" should be conducted to identify the factors noted in the standard and any deficiencies could be noted. A document covering the "quality requirements" should then be prepared and made a part of the product record or, in the new CGMP's, the Device Master Record (DMR) 21 CFR 820.181.

Note that this standard refers to the acquisition of skills which implies training. Whatever skills that will be needed for quality system personnel or line manufacturing personnel to be able to perform appropriate quality functions need to be identified and acquired. Training resources should then become a part of the general resources for the quality system. (See 21 CFR 820.25(b))

4.2.3d) *The updating, as necessary, of quality control, inspection, and testing techniques, including the development of new instrumentation;*

The requirement in 4.2.3d) may be met by preparing a single high level document or, depending on the company's Quality System structure, several middle level documents. These documents should define requirements for the periodic review of control, inspection, and testing techniques. Since each of these areas should be described in an SOP, the document should require a review of the SOP to verify a correlation between the work that is actually being done and the description in the SOP. At a minimum, this should be done annually by the personnel actually responsible for the performance of the work. Seldom used documents, such as emergency or standby procedures, could be reviewed by the supervisor who will be responsible for their implementation. This review does need to be documented, but this can be done with a simple sheet with a check-off box that states that the "work conforms to the procedure; no changes are necessary," and a second box that notes "work does not conform to the procedure; the following changes have been initiated," along with an open area that allows a written description of what modifications were made to bring the work and procedure into conformance and a space for the signature of the responsible individual. These records of SOP reviews should be held in SOP history files, specific to each SOP and arranged by SOP number, that contain records of document changes as noted in 21 CFR 820.40(b).

The document should also require a second review usually done at least once every two years for certain documents in quality and technical areas. This, second, review should compare the procedure or technique with the state of art of the applicable field. New procedures or newly available instrumentation may allow the development of a more efficient or informative technique, and this review should address this possibility and justify any decision to make or not make a change. Also, the possibility of the construction of a new testing instrument that would improve the efficiency or information level of the technique should be considered. This is especially important for those who deal with highly specialized tests that already may require the construction of special test equipment or gauges. The review should be conducted by a technically competent supervisor who is aware of the current literature in his field. The review should be written and a copy of it should be placed in the file that contains the history of the SOP as noted in 21 CFR 820.40(b).

4.2.3e) *The identification of any measurement requirement involving capability that exceeds the known state of the art, in sufficient time for the needed capability to be developed;*

In most cases the requirements of 4.2.3e) will not be a problem, as the medical products industry is well developed enough that instruments and techniques are available for most of the tests needed for a specific type of product. The author is, however, aware of at least two situations where the potency test for a product involved a difficult and laborious (therefore very expensive) animal test that precluded any sensible process control testing. The result of this "flying blind," in one case, was a highly inefficient and variable production process that required an enormous amount of effort to bring under control. All of this happened despite the availability of simple techniques that, if combined properly, could have produced a simple assay that could have replaced the animal tests at least for in-process testing. The problem here was that a review of the type required by this standard was not done, and the manufacturer was ignorant of the new developments.

This requirement can be met by a review comparing needed measurements (remember to consult the Regulatory Affairs group and, also, Marketing) to available measurement techniques. This should happen early in the device development stages to allow time for developing a method for making the measurement, if necessary, and a record of the review should become a part of the design history file (DHF).

4.3 Contract Review

4.3.1 General. *The supplier shall establish and maintain documented procedures for contract review and coordination of these activities.*

Note 9 *Channels for communication and interfaces with the customer's organization in these contract matters should be established.*

The requirements in 21 CFR 820.50 and 21 CFR 820.160 do not cover the requirements of Note 9 for either the manufacturer's suppliers or customers. The requirement in Note 9 can be satisfied by a document specifying the responsibilities for contract change control (see 4.3.3) and for communications and interfacing with the customer. Since the contract is now a document that will contain product or performance specifications and may be used as a standard for the performance of audits by the customer, it is a quality document and should be subject to formal change control with the customer possibly involved with the approval process. Since a contract is a two-party document, it would seem reasonable to involve the second party in any decisions on a proposed change.

4.3.2 Review. *Before submission of a tender, or at the acceptance of a contract or order (statement of requirement), the tender, contract, or order shall be reviewed by the supplier to ensure that:*

4.3.2a) *The requirements are adequately defined and documented; where no written statement of requirement is available for an order received by verbal means, the supplier shall ensure that the order requirements are agreed before their acceptance;*

4.3.2b) *Any differences between the contract or accepted order requirements and those in the tender are resolved;*

4.3.2c) *The supplier has the capability to meet the contract or accepted order requirements.*

These sections in 4.3.2 create the need for a document that will describe a procedure for the manufacturer to ensure that the product will meet the customer's needs and that the supplier and customer will have a mutual understanding of product requirements before the order is accepted. This will be a "Sales" document and should be prepared in cooperation with that department.

4.3.3 Amendment to Contract. *The supplier shall identify how an amendment to a contract is made and correctly transferred to the functions concerned within the supplier's organization.*

In addition to the comments made above for Note 9, the amendment to contract requirement needs to be met with a specification on how the concerned functions will be notified of contract amendments. One way would be to insert a step in the document change control protocols that would require all affected departments to participate in the approval of an amended contract. This should minimize the number of embarrassing events, such as when the Sales staff promises product qualities that manufacturing cannot provide.

4.3.4 Records. *Records of contract reviews shall be maintained (see 4.16).*

Unlike 21 CFR 820.50(b), which seems to be a function of the Purchasing Department, these contract reviews would need to be conducted by the Sales or Marketing Departments. The records themselves should be maintained by the document group created to meet the needs of 21 CFR 820.40 and Subpart M.

4.4 Design Control

4.4.4 Design Input. *Design-input requirements relating to the product, including applicable statutory and regulatory requirements, shall be identified, documented, and their selection reviewed by the supplier for adequacy. Incomplete, ambiguous, or conflicting requirements shall be resolved with those responsible for imposing those requirements.*

Design input shall take into consideration the results of any contract-review activities.

Most of this requirement is covered in 21 CFR 820.30(c), because it is understood that conflicts shall be resolved before accepting elements of design input and the later requirements for design review, verification, and validation require the resolution of conflicts. The ISO standards add a requirement that the design input should consider the results of contract review activities. As the contract review activities that are being referred to here are those between the manufacturer and the customer, the ISO requirement is basically stating that customer needs should be considered as a design input, and a mechanism for this activity needs to be in place. Section 21 CFR 820.30(c) refers to including the needs of the user and patient and also covers this requirement.

It may be argued that 21 CFR 820.30(c) includes safety as one of the *needs of the user and patient* or that it is covered in 21 CFR 820.30(f) under the *identify potential sources of harm* statement. The Design Control Guidance document clearly gives requirements for safety studies and hazard management. Therefore, except for the contract review provision, the requirements of this standard can be met within the context of 21 CFR 820.30.

4.4.5c) Design Output. *Identify those characteristics of the design that are crucial to the safe and proper functioning of the product (e.g. operating, storage, handling, maintenance, and disposal requirements).*

The preceding discussion of safety (4.4.4) from the point of view of 21 CFR 820.30(c) and (f) should be considered in 4.4.5c). Also, the Design Control Guidance document discusses the safety and hazard management required to meet the needs of 21 CFR 820.30, and the "Do It by Design" guidance document covers the requirements for Human Factors engineering. Reference to the guidance documents will provide coverage for this standard. ANSI/AAMI/ISO 13485 contains a requirement that the need for risk analysis must be evaluated during the design process, and records of any analysis performed must be maintained. These activities may be incorporated into the work on the design output or performed as a separate function of the design development team.

4.5 Document and Data Control

4.5.2c) Document and Data Approval and Issue. *This control shall ensure that: . . . Any obsolete documents retained for legal and/or knowledge-preservation purposes are suitably identified.*

There are many reasons for keeping obsolete documents available for review. However, it is not wise to have them freely available to all and to have them in a condition that makes them difficult to distinguish from current documents. 21 CFR 820.40(a) makes it clear that the document control system should have a good method for clearly identifying obsolete documents.

EN 46001:1994 (given under 4.5.1 in EN 46001) requires that the supplier should state the period for retaining obsolete documents and refers to the requirements of 4.16. The period should be at least as long as the lifetime of the device. This latter requirement can be met through compliance with 21 CFR 820.180(b) by including all documents under the definition of records.

The reference to 4.16 means that the documents that need to be retained are quality documents. The EN 46001 requirements need to be incorporated into the manufacturer's document control procedures. Given the nature of some product liability lawsuits, the manufacturer may want to specify an extended time of storage for obsolete documents rather than just for the lifetime of the device.

4.6 Purchasing

4.6.3 Purchasing Data. *Purchasing documents shall contain data clearly describing the product ordered, including where applicable:*

a) *the type, class, grade, or other precise identification.*
b) *the title or other positive identification, and applicable issues of specifications, drawings, process requirements, inspection instructions, and other relevant technical data, including requirements for approval or qualification of product, procedures, process equipment, and personnel.*
c) *the title, number, and issue of the quality-system standard to be applied.*

The supplier shall review and approve purchasing documents for adequacy of the specified requirements prior to release.

The preceding requirements may be covered under 21 CFR 820.50(b), but the ISO standard is more specific about what is expected. Thus the manufacturer who is in the process of complying with 21 CFR 820.50(b) should cover the ISO standard as well by reviewing 4.6.3 and including its requirements.

EN 46001:1994 requires the purchaser to keep copies of purchasing documents that would be important for tracing the fate of components and parts. This EN 46001 requirement is implied in 21 CFR 820.60 and 21 CFR 820.65 and can be met by including explicit statements in the documents prepared for meeting the CGMP.

4.6.4 Verification of Purchased Product

Section 4.6.4 contains two paragraphs that are somewhat different from the CGMP equivalents. Basically, the CGMP requirement in 21 CFR 820.80(a) and (b) requires verification activities relative to incoming material, but the ISO requirements apply to somewhat different situations.

4.6.4.1 Supplier Verification at Subcontractor's Premises. *Where the supplier proposes to verify purchased product at the subcontractor's premises, the supplier shall specify verification arrangements and the method of product release in the purchasing documents.*

The requirement in 4.6.4.1 applies when the manufacturer (as buyer) wishes to perform verification activities at the vendor's place of business. The requirement is that the arrangements include material acceptance/release procedures. If the manufacturer wishes to do this, purchasing documents need to be prepared to allow these activities.

4.6.4.2 Customer Verification of Subcontracted Product. *Where specified in the contract, the supplier's customer or the customer's representative shall be afforded the right to verify at the subcontractor's premises and the supplier's premises that the subcontracted product conforms to specified requirements. Such verification shall not be used by the supplier as evidence of effective control of quality by the subcontractor.*

Verification by the customer shall not absolve the supplier of the responsibility to provide acceptable product, nor shall it preclude subsequent rejection by the customer.

The manufacturer's customer may conduct verification activities on the vendor's premises as well as at the manufacturer's, if the contract so specifies. However, the customer's activities do not relieve the manufacturer from its responsibility to control the goods supplied or to monitor or assess the vendor's quality system.

In this situation, the manufacturer mainly needs to have documents that allow the manufacturer to perform vendor verification activities either independently or in cooperation with the customer. The manufacturer must review contracts with the customer as well as with the vendor to the manufacturer and should have appropriate documents available in the Sales and Purchasing departments.

In this and the preceding paragraphs, one possible approach that may result in a different set of documents is the situation where the vendor is operating a process that is being monitored under statistical process control (SPC) procedures. In these circumstances, if the vendor can provide documentation of a process that is stable and in control, the manufacturer or customer may want to consider accepting the vendor's verification activities in place of additional verification of incoming goods. This procedure will probably require audits by the manufacturer or customer to monitor the vendor's SPC operations, and periodic product testing and inspection to verify the vendor's controls. This activity could be considered as a type of in-plant verification conducted either by the manufacturer or its customer. If it is done carefully under the right circumstances, it could result in a net savings to the manufacturer and customer.

4.7 Control of Customer-Supplied Product

The supplier shall establish and maintain documented procedures for the control of verification, storage, and maintenance of customer-supplier product provided for incorporation into the supplies or for related activities. Any such product that is lost, damaged, or is otherwise unsuitable for use shall be recorded and reported to the customer (see 4.16).

Verification by the supplier does not absolve the customer of the responsibility to provide acceptable product.

If customer-supplied product is handled in the same manner as any other supplied parts or components, 21 CFR 820.80 of the CGMP should cover the verification and storage controls. The ISO standard appears to go further in requiring the control of any maintenance of the customer-supplied product. Also, there is the requirement that the customer be notified of any material that becomes unavailable for use. While it may seem natural that a manufacturer would do these things, the ISO requirements mean that these items should be specifically addressed in the manufacturer's documents.

4.8 Product Identification and Traceability

The ISO requirements would appear to be met through compliance with 21 CFR 820.60, 21 CFR 820.65, and 21 CFR 820.160, but EN 46001:1994 and ANSI/AAMI/ISO 13485:1996 added some more specific requirements:

First: Devices that are received for refurbishing must be identified and distinguished from normal production. 21 CFR 820.90(a) appears to cover this requirement, but the more specific needs should be incorporated. Manufacturers should take a broad view of refurbishing and apply this requirement to any rework, repair, or warranty work on devices that were once released, returned, and then restored to a releasable state. A document specifying a lot number series and specific handling and identification instructions for these refurbished devices should meet this requirement. The provisions of 21 CFR 820.200 could be extended to cover refurbishing.

Second: For implantable devices the traceability must be extended to all components and material used in manufacturing. Also the manufacturer must be able to trace the records of the environmental conditions that could adversely affect the performance of the device. The first part of this requirement should not be difficult to meet, as most prudent device manufacturers already provide for the traceability of raw material and component lots through to the final product. The insertion of requirements for recording lot numbers of parts and components in manufacturing lot records should meet this standard.

The second part of this requirement is captured in 21 CFR 820.70(c) for all devices subject to the CGMP. Tracking via lot numbers and production dates should allow a determination of environmental conditions at the times when the device was under the manufacturer's control. Manufacturers should be very careful about this requirement. Many manufacturers do perform environmental monitoring, but it is often done in a fashion that divorces it from the processing that occurs. Consequently it is quite common to find manufacturing taking place at a time when the environment in the manufacturing area was out of specifications. The mechanism by which environmental monitoring data will be used to control manufacturing activities, needs to be clearly specified.

4.9 Process Control

All of the parts of this ANSI/ISO/ASQC 9001:1994 section and the EN 46001:1994 appear to be covered by the CGMP, but the EN 46001 section contains adjustments to requirements for products that are cleaned before use. Basically, the manufacturer is relieved of personnel and environmental controls if the product is to be cleaned before sterilization and use. Manufacturers subject to the CGMP will not want to take advantage of these provisions as they are actually less than what is required by the CGMP. Keeping the environmental and personnel controls required by the CGMP will simply exceed EN 46001 requirements and should not result in a violation. The situation appears to be different in ANSI/AAMI/ISO 13485:1996 where devices that are supplied in a nonsterile condition and intended for sterilization before use should have requirements for environmental control added to their specifications. ANSI/AAMI/ISO 13485 contains several process control standards related to personnel, environmental control, cleanliness, maintenance, installation and software. These requirements are covered in various parts of the Quality System regulations, not necessarily just the parts related to process controls.

EN 46001, 4.9.2 specifically requires that for special processes (one whose outcome cannot be assessed by subsequent evaluation) the quality records must identify the date of performance, the work instruction used, and the identity of the personnel executing the process. Note that these processes should have been the subject of process validations during the development phase.

This section also contains a specific requirement for manufacturers of sterile medical devices, but any manufacturer of such a device working under CGMP rules will already be complying with its requirements, which are for validation of the sterilization process and recording of the control parameters during the sterilization.

4.10 Inspection and Testing

4.10.2.2 *In determining the amount and nature of receiving inspection, consideration shall be given to the amount of control exercised at the subcontractor's premises and the recorded evidence of conformance provided.*

Although this is normally done by CGMP compliant companies, it is not so clearly stated in the CGMP requirements. These requirements should be incorporated into the manufacturer's thinking on 21 CFR 820.50(a)(2).

4.10.2.3 *Where incoming product is released for urgent production purposes prior to verification, it shall be positively identified and recorded (see 4.16) in order to permit immediate recall and replacement in the event of nonconformity to specified requirements.*

Manufacturers often have a mechanism for using incoming material that has not been officially released (usually by a QA or QC group) for use in manufacturing. The ISO requirement for positive identification and recording of this status means that a formal procedure that incorporates "flags" or other notices should be created to cover this situation. This requirement could be added to documents covering 21 CFR 820.80, 21 CFR 820.86, or 21 CFR 820.90(b). In some companies, this advanced release for urgent production needs is almost a routine process and is handled without any special paperwork with the QA or QC group being left to catch up as they can. This practice must be improved to comply with the ISO requirements, and may, from time to time, draw fire from FDA inspectors, especially if it really becomes a routine practice. This type of behavior is usually a sign of poor management or of an attitude that QA or QC functions only impede manufacturing and have little value to offer the company.

4.11 Control of Inspection, Measuring, and Test Equipment

4.11.2 Control Procedure.   The supplier shall: a) determine the measurements to be made and the accuracy required, and select the appropriate inspection, measuring, and test equipment that is capable of the necessary accuracy and precision;

The control procedure information should be placed in the Device Master Record under 21 CFR 820.181(c), as it provides additional details for that part of the CGMP. This section might also be interpreted as requiring validation of the measurement processes to at least demonstrate the needed level of accuracy and precision. Good Quality Management should already have these considerations included as part of the product development process under design control, but in many firms, these activities are a matter of chance, not planning.

The supplier shall: f) assess and document the validity of previous inspection and test results when inspection, measuring, and test equipment is found to be out of calibration;

Many firms already have a requirement that, when an instrument or other measuring device is found to be out of calibration, all results must be checked back to the date when the instrument or device was last known to be functioning properly. It is at these times that a good test control material will prove its worth. This action needs to be written into a QA or Metrology procedure under a section covering actions to be taken if an instrument of device fails to pass calibration checks.

The supplier shall: g) ensure that the environmental conditions are suitable for the calibrations, inspections, measurements, and tests being carried out;

This section is a bit different from 21 CFR 820.72(b), which appears to be the corresponding CGMP section. Basically, it means that environmental conditions must be right for the performance of the activity. This means that the group charged with the performance of the test should first determine if environmental factors can affect the outcome of the test. If so, then they should make arrangements for the performance of the test under suitable conditions with monitoring, if necessary, to verify the presence of the proper environment for the activity that will be conducted. All of this, of course, should be documented, including any determination that environment is not a factor.

4.13 Control of Nonconforming Product

4.13.2 Review and Disposition. The responsibility for review and authority for the disposition of nonconforming product shall be defined.

Nonconforming product shall be reviewed in accordance with documented procedures. It may be:

a) reworked to meet the specified requirements,
b) accepted with or without repair by concession,
c) regraded for alternative applications or
d) rejected or scrapped.

Where required by contract, the proposed use or repair of product (see 4.13.2b) which does not conform to specified requirements shall be reported for concession to the customer or customer's representative. The description of the nonconformity that has been accepted, and of repairs, shall be recorded to denote the actual condition (4.16).

Repaired and/or reworked product shall be reinspected in accordance with the quality plan and/or documented procedures.

This whole section, including the section in EN 46001:1994, is actually covered in 21 CFR 820.90. Paragraph 820.90(a) indirectly discusses a Material Review Board that will be responsible for the reviews and disposition of all nonconforming material. However, the ISO standard specifically covers the four methods of disposition listed above, while the CGMP regulation is not as specific. Also, the ISO document refers to notifications to customers based on contractual requirements. The CGMP approach would be to say that contractual requirements will always be met, and the parties to the contract may agree to any reporting requirements that they wish to employ.

ANSI/AAMI/ISO 13485:1996 contains a statement that the manufacturer must ensure that nonconforming product is accepted by concession only if regulatory requirements are met, and the identities of the people authorizing the concessions are recorded. Other requirements of ANSI/AAMI/ISO 13485:1996 are met in 21 CFR 820.90(b)(2).

4.14 Corrective and Preventive Action

4.14.3 Preventive Action.   *The procedures for preventive action shall include:*

a) *the use of appropriate sources of information such as processes and work operations which affect product quality, concessions, audit results, quality records, service reports, and customer complaints to detect, analyze, and eliminate potential causes of nonconformities;*
b) *determination of the steps needed to deal with any problems requiring preventive action;*
c) *initiation of preventive action and application of controls to ensure that it is effective;*
d) *confirmation that relevant information on actions taken is submitted for management review (see 4.1.3).*

The difference here is in the requirement that information be submitted for management review. The CGMP requires documentation of the actions, and that carries with it the implication that management review has or will occur. For compliance with the ISO requirement, a clear instruction that information on the actions must be submitted for management review should be incorporated into a standard operating procedure, along with a requirement to record the results of the management review.

ANSI/AAMI/ISO 13485:1996 states that the manufacturer must establish and maintain a documented feedback system for the early detection of quality problems. The information obtained from this feedback system should be used for corrective or preventive actions. All sources of feedback information should be considered and a documented review of the information gathered shall be performed periodically.

EN 46001:1994 adds the requirement that the monitoring and review system incorporate any required post marketing monitoring system. Also, the review and monitoring must be handled by a designated individual. EN 46001 further states that when an investigation finds that activities at a remote location were at least partially responsible for a complaint, a copy of the complaint report must be sent to that location. The CGMP (see 21 CFR 820.198(f)) requires that a copy of all pertinent complaints be accessible to the actual manufacturing organization.

En 46001 expects the manufacturer to have procedures for issuing advisory notices in addition to being able to recall medical devices. Both of these activities mean that the sales department needs to be aware of which customers possess the devices (see 21 CFR 820.160) and also be able to issue general notices in trade journals to inform any device owners whose addresses may not be known to the Sales personnel.

4.15 Handling, Storage, Packaging, Preservation, and Delivery

EN 46001:1994 contains a provision requiring procedures (if appropriate) for handling used product to avoid contamination of other devices or the manufacturing environment. This should be considered and added, if necessary, to any statements made in response to 21 CFR 820.150.

4.15.4 Packaging. *The supplier shall control packing, packaging, and marking processes (including materials used) to the extent necessary to ensure conformation to specified requirements.*

The marking process is covered by the CGMP if it can be considered to be a label. In ANSI/AAMI/ISO 13485:1996, Note 6 states that "marking" is interpreted to mean labeling, so the GMPC is applicable. ANSI/AAMI/ISO 13485 contains a specific requirement for recording the identities of the people who conduct the labeling operation on an implantable device.

EN 46001:1994 expresses concern over the maintenance of sterility and requires a mechanism to reveal opening or other exposure of inner surfaces if the product is such that only the inner surface of the packaging or device needs to be sterile. This may add a factor to be considered as a part of the design input in 21 CFR 820.30(c) and 21 CFR 820.160.

For labeling operations, EN 46001 requires the manufacturer to record the identity of the operators who do the labeling and not just the person who inspected the labels as required in 21 CFR 820.120(d).

4.15.6 Delivery. *The supplier shall arrange for the protection of the quality of product after final inspection and test. Where contractually specified, this protection shall be extended to include delivery to destination.*

Once again, the initial reaction is to say that, "Of course we will do whatever is contractually specified," and the manufacturer should ensure the proper handling of the product during distribution and shipment to the final destination. (This is one of the reasons for doing shipping validations.) However, to ensure ISO compliance a statement to cover the above requirement should be entered into the documents covering 21 CFR 820.160. Also for tracked devices, meeting the provisions of 21 CFR 821 will provide an opportunity to insert the ISO requirements.

ANSI/AAMI/ISO 13485:1996 requires that the name and address of the shipping package consignee must be added to the quality records for implantable devices.

4.16 Control of Quality Records. *The supplier shall establish and maintain documented procedures for identification, collection, indexing, access, filing, storage, maintenance, and disposition of quality records.*

Quality records shall be maintained to demonstrate conformance to specified requirements and the effective operation of the quality system. Pertinent quality records from the subcontractor shall be an element of these data.

All quality records shall be legible and shall be stored and re-tained in such a way that they are readily retrievable in facilities that provide a suitable environment to prevent damage or deterioration and to prevent loss. Retention times of quality records shall be es-tablished and recorded. Where agreed contractually, quality records shall be made available for evaluation by the customer or the cus-tomer's representative for an agreed period.

Note 19 *Records may be in the form of any type of media, such as hard copy or electronic media.*

The main problem here is in the list of specific documented pro-cedures that the ISO standard lists. The requirement for obtaining and maintaining pertinent quality records from a vendor also needs to be defined. Some of these actions will already be required by documents that address the device CGMP. All that is then needed is to review these documents to make certain that clear statements that satisfy the requirements are made. For instance the document that defines the procedures for identifying quality records should also have a statement on how pertinent quality records from the vendor will be identified and requested. Also, certain documents related to installation (21 CFR 820.170) and servicing (21 CFR 820.200) need to be obtained from third parties.

EN 46001:1994 adds a requirement that the Device History Record (21 CFR 820.184) should be reviewed and authorized. ANSI/AAMI/ISO 13485:1996 states that the batch record should be verified and authorized.

4.18 Training

EN 46001:1994 appears to allow for supervision by a trained person for work on special processes or special environments by personnel who are untrained. The CGMP (21 CFR 820.25(b)) requires training, and special environments are covered in 21 CFR 820.70(d), so this is probably not an important issue. The main problem here lies in the definition of "trained person." The manufacturer will want to give some thought to this term. This definition could become very important in the event of an accident or other costly event that may arise from insufficient or inappropriate training.

BIBLIOGRAPHY

The following is a list of the documents that have been used in the preceding discussions on the CGMPs. They are listed by their commonly used shortened names or by their full titles, if no commonly used shortened name is known, but their full titles are also given. Unless otherwise stated, all of these documents may be obtained from the CDRH (DSMA, FDA). ISO documents are available through various agencies that maintain standards and also several private companies that specialize in providing documents to the public.

Some of the following documents are not fully discussed in the text and are incorporated mainly by reference. The manufacturer will probably wish to obtain all of these documents as useful guidelines for its Quality Systems department.

ANSI/AAMI/ISO 13485:1996: Quality Systems—Medical Devices—Supplementary requirements to ISO 9001.

ANSI/ISO/ASQC A8402-1994: Quality Management and Quality Assurance—Vocabulary. Adopted as an American National Standard on Feb. 6, 1995.

ANSI/ISO/ASQC 9001:1994 also EN 29001 and BS 5750, part 1: Quality Systems—Model for Quality Assurance in Design/Development, Production, Installation, and Servicing.

CGMP Quality System regulations: Title 21 Code of Federal Regulations, Part 820 (eff. 6-1-97) in its entirety.

Critical device list: Federal Register, March 17, 1988, and 21 CFR 809.10(a)(9).

Design Control Guidance: Design Control Guidance for Medical Device Manufacturers.

Do It by Design (Risk Management Guidance): Do It By Design: An introduction to Human Factors in Medical Devices.

EN 46001:1994: Specification for Application of EN 29001 (BS 5750 : Part 1) to the Manufacture of Medical Devices.

Environmental Control Classifications: U.S. Federal Standard 209E (available through the General Services Administration).

Fair Packaging and Labeling Act

FDCA: Food Drugs and Cosmetics Act, sections 201 and 502.

ISO . . .: The following ISO standards provide guidelines in certain areas, and the manufacturer will wish to obtain those parts that will be useful. ISO 9000-1 and 9000-2 are general guidelines for the application of ANSI/ISO/ASQC 9001, 9002, and 9003; ISO 9000-3 covers software; ISO 9000-4 covers dependability management; ISO 9004-1 and 10002 are useful for quality systems and quality management guidelines; ISO 9004-3 discusses processed materials; ISO 9004-4, 10005 and 10006 are general quality assurance guidelines; ISO 10011 requires three parts to cover quality auditing; ISO 10012 requires two parts to cover the quality assurance of measuring equipment; and ISO 10015 discusses education and training requirements.

ISO 10013: Guidelines for Developing Quality Manuals.

ISO/CD 14971: Medical Devices—Risk Management— Application of Risk Analysis to Medical Devices.

Medical Device Reporting (MDR): 21 CFR 803 and 21 CFR 804.

prEN 724: Guidance on the Application of EN 29001 and EN 46001 and of EN 29002 and EN 46002 for nonactive medical devices.

prEN 928: Guidance on the Application of EN 29001/EN 46001 and EN 29002/EN 46002 for the *in vitro* diagnostic industry.

prEN 50103: Guidance on the application of EN 29001 and EN 46001 and of EN 29002 and EN 46002 for the active (including active implantable) medical device industry.

Process Validation Guidelines: Guidelines on General Principles of Process Validation (available through CDER).

Quality Systems Manual: Medical Device Quality Systems Manual: A small entity compliance guide. First edition, December 1996 (HHS Publication FDA 97-4179).

Quality System regulations: Title 21 Code of Federal Regulations, Part 820 (eff. 6-1-97) in its entirety.

Radiation Control for Health and Safety Act

Risk Management Guidance: ISO/CD 14971, "Medical Devices— Risk Management—Application of Risk Analysis to Medical Devices."

Sampling Plans: Military Standards 105E and 414E (recently reissued as ANSI/ASQ documents).

Software validation guidance: There are four documents: Application of the Medical Device GMP's to Computerized Devices and Manufacturing Processes; Reviewer Guidance for Computer Controlled Medical Devices Undergoing 510(k) Review; Military Specification MIL-S-52779A; and Standard for Software Quality Assurance Plan, IEEE Std 730-1984.

Working Draft: Working Draft of the CGMP Final Rule, Federal Register, Oct. 7, 1996 (61 FR 52601).

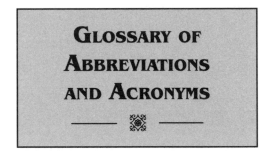

GLOSSARY OF ABBREVIATIONS AND ACRONYMS

510(k)—FDCA 510(k): Premarket Notification for Medical Devices.

ANSI—American National Standards Institute.

ASQ—American Society for Quality; formerly the ASQC, American Society for Quality Control.

BSI—British Standards Institute. A good source for English versions of European standards.

CAD/CAM—Computer Assisted Design/ Computer Assisted Manufacturing.

CAR—Corrective Action Request, usually results from the finding of a major deficiency.

CAT—Corrective Action Team, often referred to redundantly as a CAT team. Usually formed to act on a CAR.

CBER—Center for Biologics Evaluation and Research.

CCB—Change Control Board.

CDER—Center for Drugs Evaluation and Research.

CDRH—Center for Devices and Radiological Health. The division of FDA primarily responsible for medical devices.

CEN—European Committee for Standardization.

CENELEC—European Committee for Electrotechnical Standardization.

CEO—Chief Executive Officer.

CFR—Code of Federal Regulations. References are made in the form: 21 CFR 820.30, which stands for Title 21, Code of Federal Regulations, part 820, paragraph 30. There are also subparagraphs, etc.

CGMP—Current Good Manufacturing Practices, same as GMP.

CPM—Critical Path Method (not counts per minute).

CQA—Certified Quality Auditor. A certification awarded by the ASQ.

CQE—Certified Quality Engineer. A certification awarded by the ASQ.

CRE—Certified Reliability Engineer. A certification awarded by the ASQ.

CSA—Canadian Standards Association.

DHF—Design History File.

DHR—Device History Record.

DMR—Device Master Record.

DOE—Design of Experiments.

DSMA—Division of Small Manufacturer's Assistance. A part of CDRH. Often referred to as "Disma."

EN—European Standard.

FDA—Food and Drug Administration (not Federal Drug Administration).

FIFO—First-in, first-out.

FMEA—Failure Mode Effect Analysis.

FR—Federal Register. References are usually made by date of publication or in the form: 61 FR 10034, which stands for Federal Register, Volume 61, page 10034.

FTA—Fault Tree Analysis.

GLP—Good Laboratory Practices. Usually applied to preclinical safety studies (21 CFR 58).

GMP—Good Manufacturing Practices; same as CGMP.

HVAC—Heating, Ventilation, Air Conditioning.

IDE—Investigational Device Exemption.

IQ—Installation Qualification.

ISO—International Organization for Standardization (not International Standards Organization).

ISO/CD—ISO Committee Draft (supersedes an ISO/DIS).

ISO/DIS—ISO discussion document.

KGB—Committee of State Security.

MEF—MDR Event File.

MDR—Medical Device Reporting.

MRB—Materials Review Board.

OQ—Operational Qualification.

PERT—Program Evaluation and Review Technique.

PMA—Premarket Approval Application.

PQ—Process Qualification.

QA—Quality Assurance.

QC—Quality Control.

QFD—Quality Function Deployment.

QM—Quality Manual.

QSR—Quality System Records. Do not confuse this with Quality System regulations or Quality System requirements.

QS—Quality Systems.

R & D—Research and Development.

RAB—Registrar Accreditation Board. Associated with the ASQ, it accredits ISO registrars and auditors in the United States.

SPC—Statistical Process Control.

U.S.C.—United States Code. Codification of federal laws. References follow the same pattern as the CFR; this part of the authority for the GMPs is given in 21 U.S.C. 351 (Title 21, United States Code, section 351).

UL—Underwriters Laboratory.

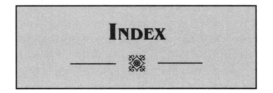

INDEX